Oxytocin and Health

Edited by Wei Wu
and Ifigenia Kostoglou-Athanassiou

Published in London, United Kingdom

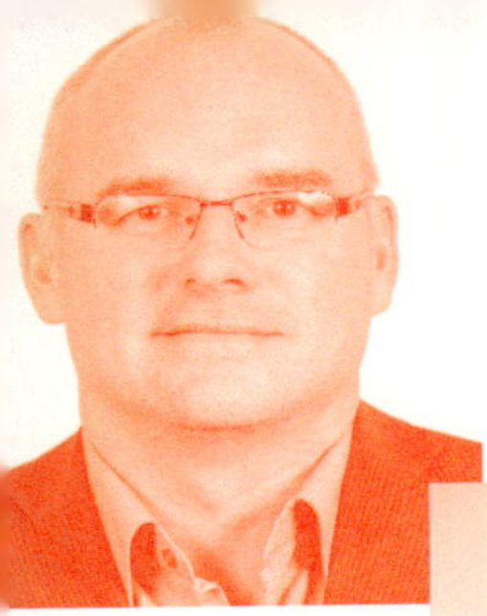
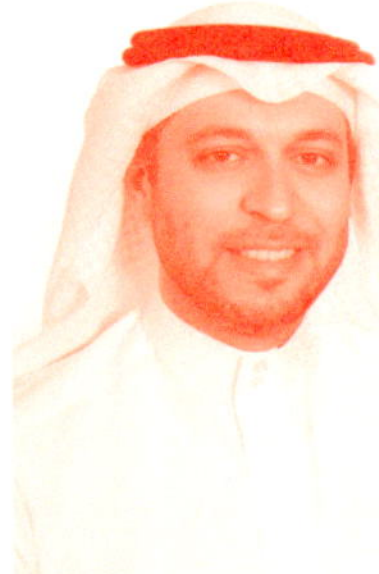
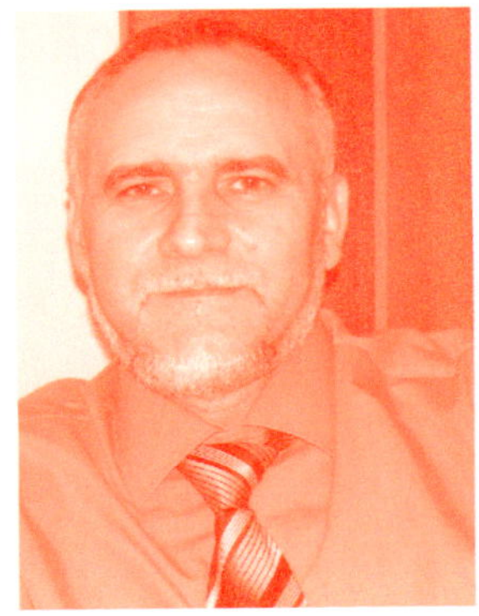
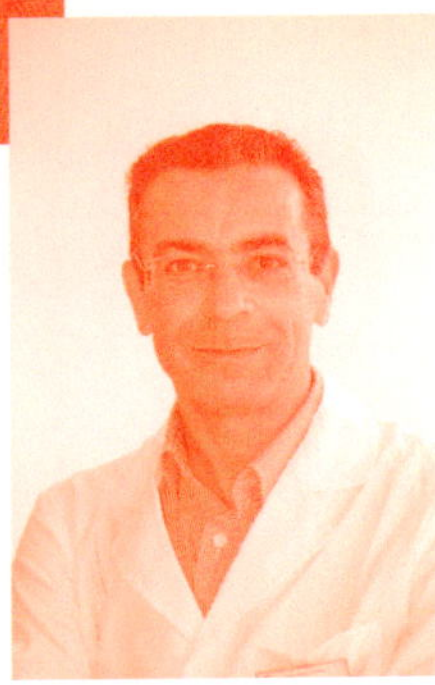
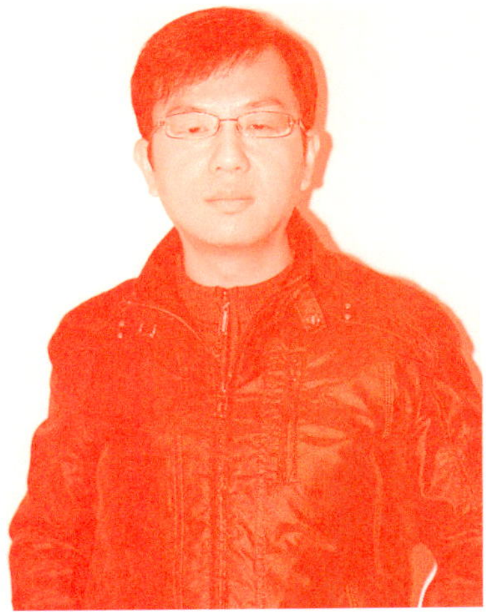
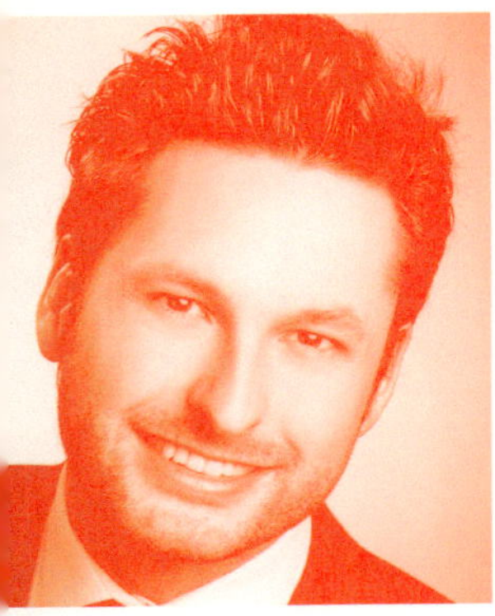
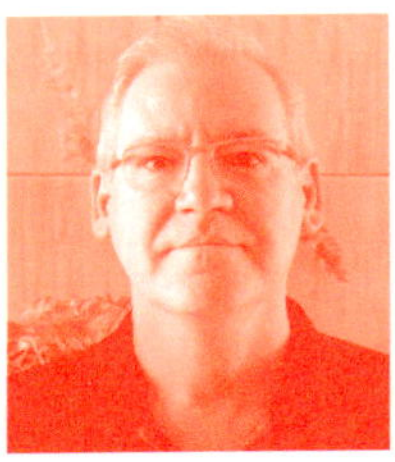

IntechOpen

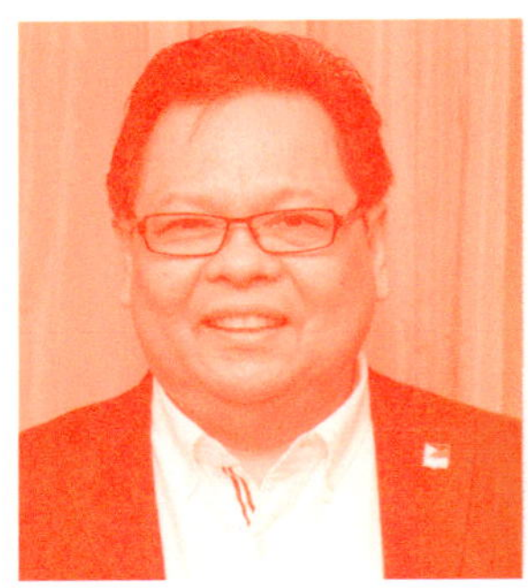
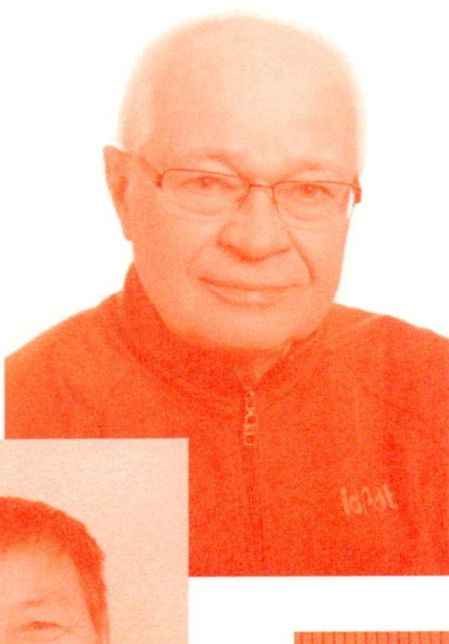
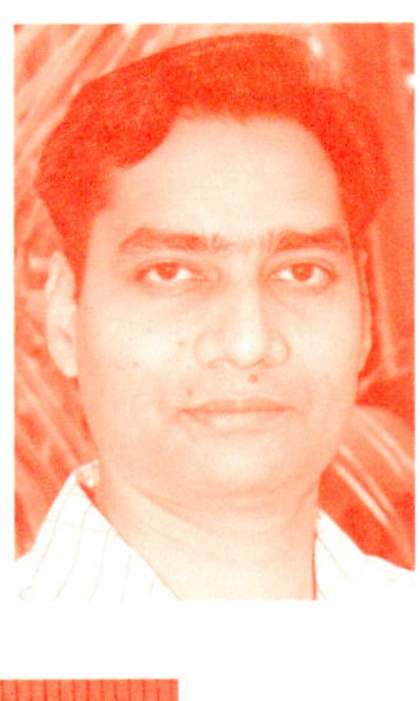
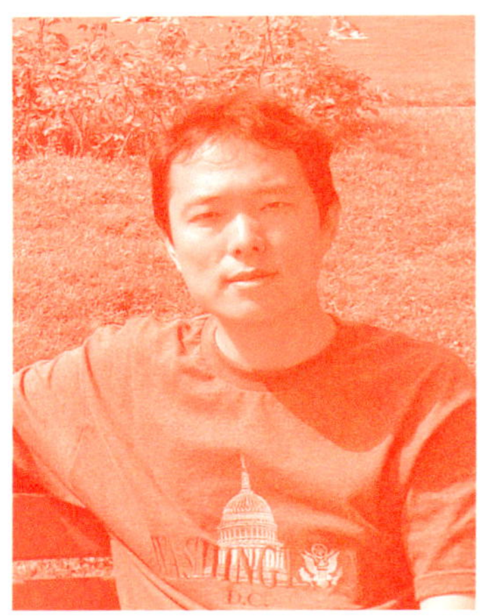
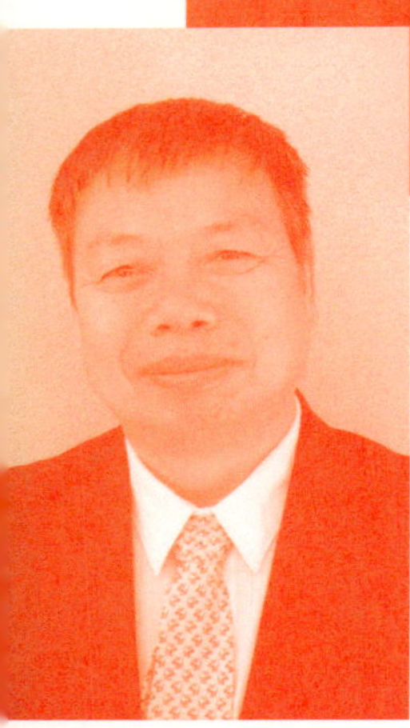
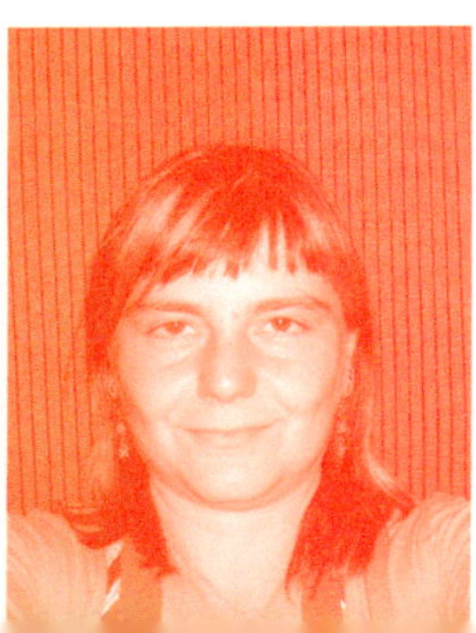

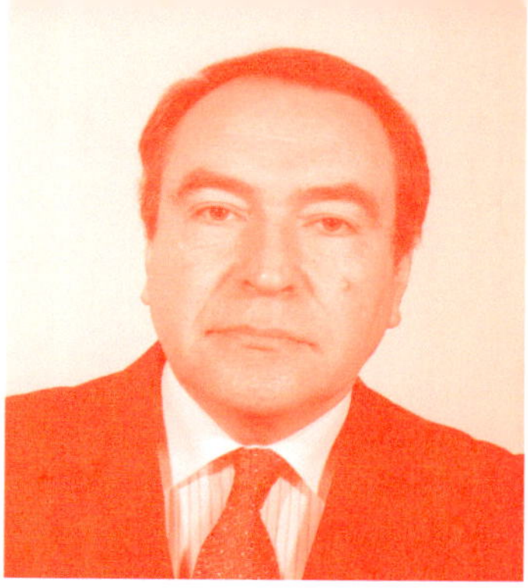
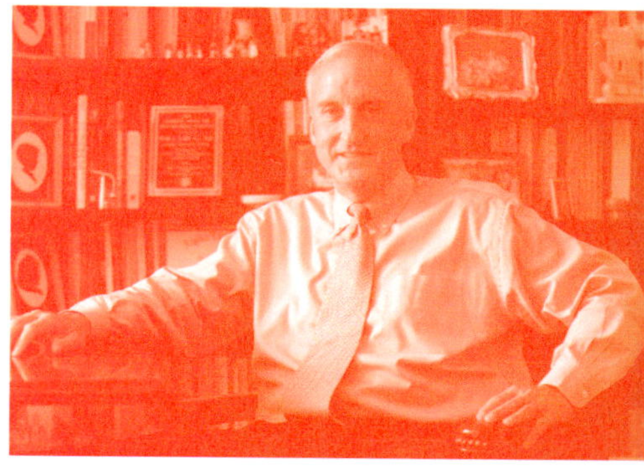
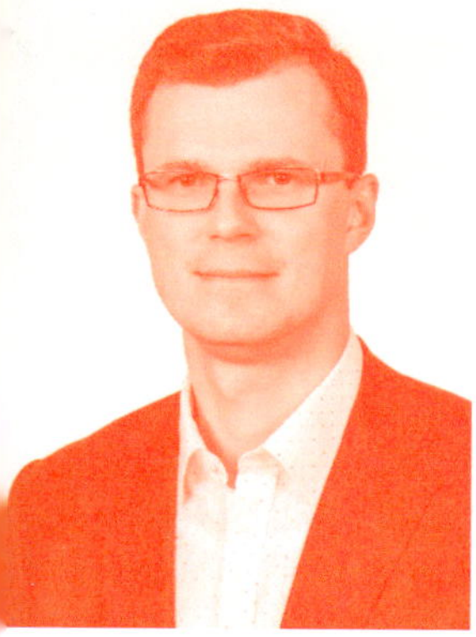
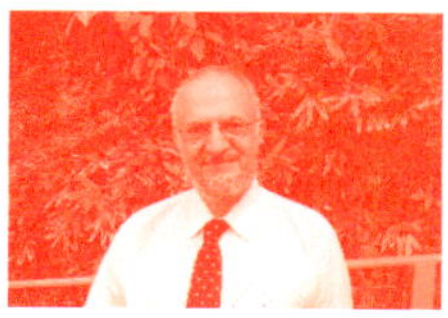
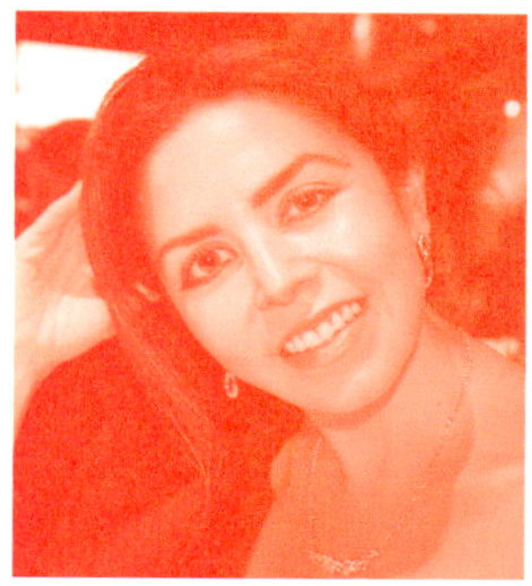

Supporting open minds since 2005

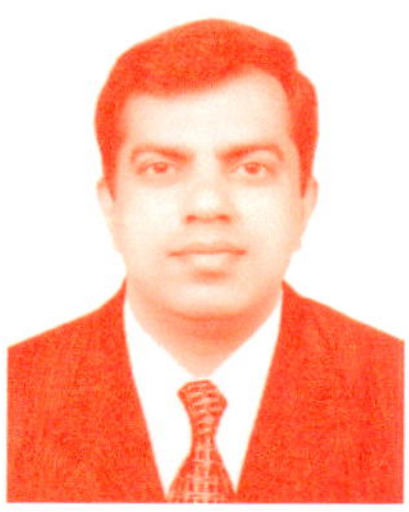
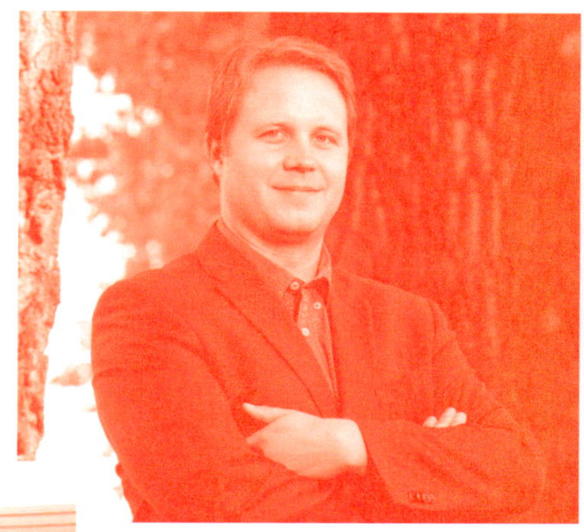
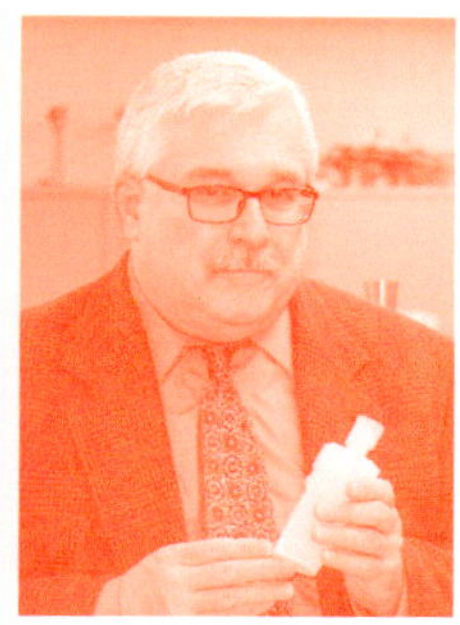
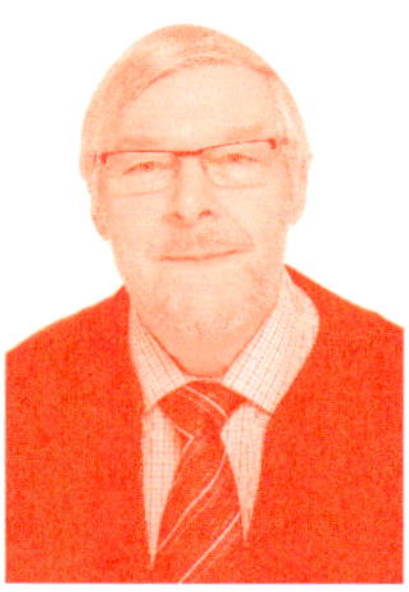
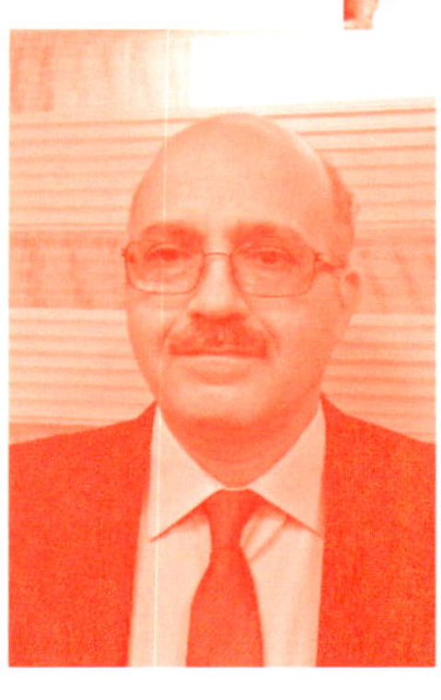
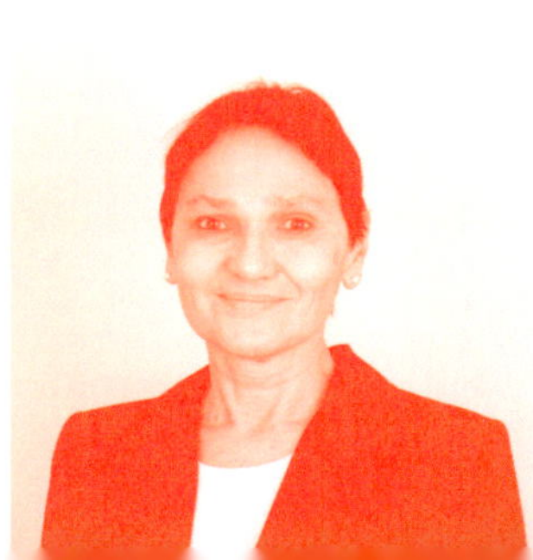
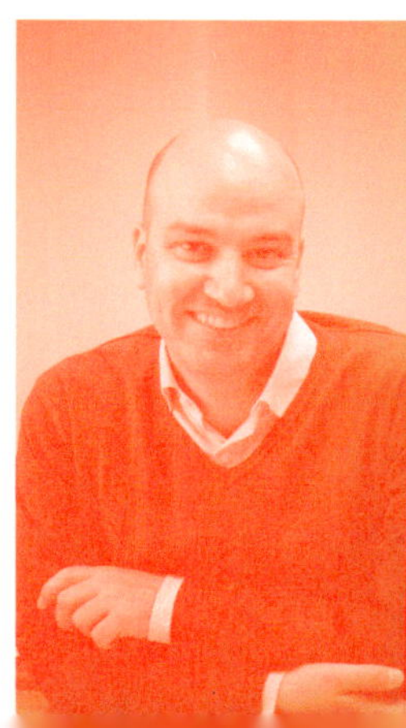

Oxytocin and Health
http://dx.doi.org/10.5772/intechopen.92479
Edited by Wei Wu and Ifigenia Kostoglou-Athanassiou

Contributors
Qiuqin Tang, Haiwen Yu, Wei Wu, Yiwen Lu, Yuting Cheng, Oytun Erbas, Ilknur Altuntas, Guillermo Osorio Revilla, Veera C.S.R Chittepu, Poonam Kalhotra, Tzayhri Gallardo-Velázquez, Katherine K.M. Stavropoulos, Elizabeth Baker, Rosa Fernandez, Karla Ramírez, Enrique Delgado Zayas, Esther Gómez Gil, Isabel Esteva, Antonio Guillamon, Eduardo Pásaro, Chitose Orikasa, Verena Nold, Kelly Allers, Neeru Bhatt

First published in London, United Kingdom, 2021 by IntechOpen
IntechOpen is the global imprint of INTECHOPEN LIMITED, registered in England and Wales, registration number: 11086078, 5 Princes Gate Court, London, SW7 2QJ, United Kingdom
Printed in Croatia

British Library Cataloguing-in-Publication Data
A catalogue record for this book is available from the British Library

Additional hard and PDF copies can be obtained from orders@intechopen.com

Oxytocin and Health
Edited by Wei Wu and Ifigenia Kostoglou-Athanassiou
p. cm.
Print ISBN 978-1-83969-137-9
Online ISBN 978-1-83969-138-6
eBook (PDF) ISBN 978-1-83969-139-3

For EU product safety concerns:
IN TECH d.o.o., Prolaz Marije Krucifikse Kozulić 3, 51000 Rijeka, Croatia, info@intechopen.com or visit our website at intechopen.com.

Meet the editors

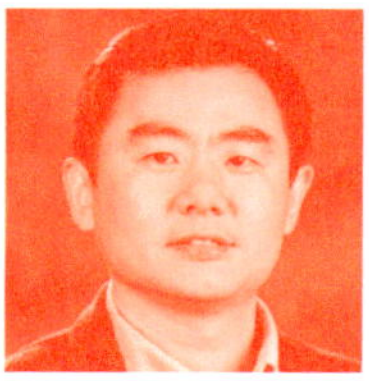

Dr. Wei Wu is an associate professor and associate department chair in the Department of Toxicology, Nanjing Medical University, China, where he received his Ph.D. in Toxicology in 2012. He was a guest researcher at the National Institute of Environmental Health Sciences (NIEHS) between 2017 and 2018. Dr. Wu is a member of different national and international societies in the fields of human reproduction and toxicology. He has received awards from many national societies for the originality and quality of his projects. Dr. Wu has authored seventy-two peer-reviewed papers in international journals, edited four books, and collaborated on ten others. He is also a reviewer for ninety-three journals. Dr. Wu has eleven patents to his credit and has participated in the organization of three international conferences.

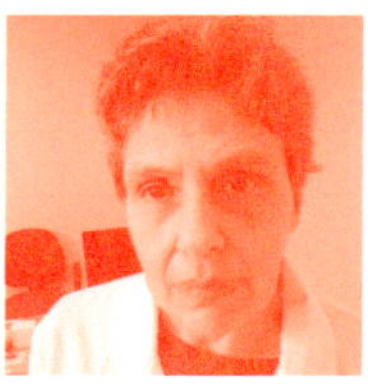

Dr. Ifigenia Kostoglou-Athanassiou was born in Thessaloniki, Greece. She is an endocrinologist who graduated from the Medical School, Aristotle University of Thessaloniki, Greece. She obtained an MD from the University of Athens Medical School, and a Ph.D. from the University of London. Her areas of research include breast cancer, neuroendocrinology, melatonin, thyroid cancer, vitamin D, and autoimmune diseases. She has won several awards for her research. Dr. Kostoglou-Athanassiou has published numerous papers and book chapters. Currently, she works as a consultant endocrinologist and head of the Endocrine Department, Asclepeion Hospital, Voula, Athens, Greece.

Contents

Preface

Oxytocin, an important neuropeptide, exerts a wide influence on the central nervous system and peripheral tissues. It regulates a range of physiologic actions in mammals other than assisting parturition and lactation functions. Oxytocin and its receptor signaling mechanism have emerged as a pathway for the treatment of endocrine disorders. This book focuses on oxytocin and health, from the aspects of molecular and structure activity, physiological and pathological functions, and clinical applications.

Chapter 1 discusses oxytocin in pregnancy as well as its clinical applications. It explores the link between oxytocin and pregnancy in three aspects: physiology, ethology, and clinical application.

Chapter 2 discusses the molecular aspects and structure activity relationship of oxytocin agonists and antagonists' role in health. This chapter outlines the phenotype characteristics of the receptor agonists and antagonists in various diseases like diabetes, obesity, and cardiovascular and immune-related diseases.

Chapter 3 includes a comprehensive study about oxytocin and its physiological and pathological functions, which makes it a potential target for drug therapy. Oxytocin can be a potential avenue for the treatment of endocrine disorders such as obesity, diabetes mellitus, and associated disorders.

Chapter 4 outlines the chemical properties of oxytocin and the neuroprotective effects of the oxytocin hormone. Oxytocin can affect the course of the disease and is promising in the treatment of neurodegenerative disorders due to its therapeutic properties and benefits.

Chapter 5 discusses combining oxytocin administration with behavioral interventions to improve social-communicative outcomes for children with an autism spectrum disorder.

Chapter 6 reviews the regulation of morphological and functional aspects of sexual dimorphism in the brain. This chapter addresses and focuses largely on the role of sex-dependent differences in the brain and their crucial functions in animal models.

Chapter 7 covers the implication of estrogens and steroid receptor coactivators in the genetic basis of gender incongruence. This chapter also discusses the candidate genes for gender incongruence.

Chapter 8 overviews the consequences of chronic stress on the psycho-immune-neuro-energy (PINE) system. Within the PINE network, glucocorticoids are the universal messengers that regulate overall physiology jointly with cytokines, neurotransmitters, and energy status.

Many individuals made this book a reality. The completion of this book would not have been possible without the efforts of numerous contributors. I would like to thank Ms. Mia Vulovic at IntechOpen for her strong support from the inception to completion of this book. I would also like to acknowledge my coauthors for their efforts.

Wei Wu
Department of Toxicology,
School of Public Health,
Nanjing Medical University,
China

Ifigenia Kostoglou-Athanassiou
Department of Endocrinology,
Asclepeion Hospital,
Voula, Athens, Greece

Chapter 1

Oxytocin and Pregnancy

Haiwen Yu, Yuting Cheng, Yiwen Lu, Wei Wu and Qiuqin Tang

Abstract

Oxytocin, an important neuropeptide, exerts a wide influence on the central nervous system and the peripheral tissues. In the central nervous system, the oxytocin gene expression is mainly shown to be present in neurons in the hypothalamic paraventricular and supraoptic nuclei. Oxytocin gene also transcribes in the peripheral tissues such as uterus, placenta, and amnion. Oxytocin receptors can be founded in many tissues in humans, like the uterine, ovary, testis, kidney, and so on. And just in the same tissue, due to the variation of physiology factors, the amount of oxytocin changes a lot. Oxytocin secretion is closely linked with pregnancy advancing. During labor, the contractions of uterine smooth muscles and oxytocin secretion are inseparable. Moreover, oxytocin is also responsible for stimulating milk ejection after parturition. Oxytocin is associated with many diseases. Poor regulation of oxytocin may cause postpartum depression and infantile autism. In terms of physiology, fatal heart failure and gestational hypertension are concerned with oxytocin level. In this chapter, we will discuss the oxytocin in pregnancy as well as its clinical applications.

Keywords: ovary, oxytocin, pregnancy, parturition, reproductive tissues, testis, uterine

1. Introduction

Oxytocin (OT) is crucial to pregnancy which exerts an important physiological influence on the central nervous system and the peripheral tissues [1]. Some findings suggest that OT secretion is closely linked with pregnancy advancing. And during labor, the contractions of uterine smooth muscles and OT, as well as its receptors, are inseparable. Moreover, OT is also responsible for stimulating milk ejection after parturition.

OT receptors founded in many tissues in humans, like the uterine, ovary, testis, kidney, and so on, are also important to pregnancy. Due to the variation of physiological factors during pregnancy, just in the same tissue, the amount of OT receptors differs a lot. Further studies illustrate that the oxytocin receptor (OTR) expression appears to be regulated at the transcriptional level [2].

And as such, OT disorder is associated with many diseases. To behavioral effects, poor regulation of OT may cause postpartum depression and autism spectrum disorders. In terms of physiology, premature delivery and dysmenorrhea are concerned with OT levels. Therefore, the clinical application of OT is also worthy of attention.

2. Oxytocin and its receptors in physiology

2.1 Male reproductive tissues

OT plays a physiological role in the male reproductive tract across species. In the human [3], OT messenger RNA (mRNA) and peptide itself are distributed in the testis where OTR has also been identified in the Leydig cells and Sertoli cells. But it is important to note that the species-specific differences in the case of the localization of the OT system in the male reproductive tract. For instance, in normal mice, testicular OT mRNA level is low to be detected while cattle have relatively high levels of OT mRNA in their testes [4]. OTR distribution characteristics are similar to the OT. The OT receptors were localized in the testis of the rats [4]. However, in the tammar wallaby, the mesotocin receptor gene and protein, which are highly homologous to the OT receptor, are not expressed in the testis, but in the prostate gland [5].

OT in the male reproductive system is not limited to the testis, the paracrine mode has high similarity with the OT secretion style in female reproductive tissues. Significant amounts of the peptide can be detected in the prostate and epididymis [6]. In the human, OT appears to exist in testis, epididymis, and prostate.

Testicular OT may have a role to play in the reproductive processes of the male by influencing the production of gonadal steroids. OT was found to stimulate testosterone production in mice [7], as well as in goats and pre-pubertal rats [8, 9]. In cell experiments of rat Leydig cells, OT also has the foundation to stimulate testosterone production [10]. But this effect remains controversial. In other purified Leydig cells research, no significant effect was observed [11]. Meanwhile, as well known, testosterone is an important agonist of ejaculation. So, OT may play an indirect role in the physiological process of male reproduction by gonadal steroids, especially testosterone.

What's more, the crosstalk between OT and vasopressin is also worthy of attention. In different species [12], the crosstalk phenomenon has been found [12]. Current research findings suggest that the affinity of OT to both OTR and vasopressin receptors is similar whereas OT has a higher affinity to its receptor than to vasopressin receptors. Vasopressin might also have an important effect on OT-mediated contractility in human myometrium and the ejaculation related tissues (prostatic urethra, bladder neck, and ejaculatory duct) of rats and rabbits [13].

Nevertheless, the classic roles of both peptides are still preserved; where OT is associated with contractile effects in both genders (ejaculation in men and uterus contraction in women) and social behaviors whereas vasopressin is closely related to water homeostasis and blood pressure regulation. OT acting through AVP-receptors and its receptor, which may explain some observed OT side effects, like headache and dizziness. This interaction between OT and vasopressin may also explain why vasopressin while showing similar contractibility to OT in the male reproductive tract, may also cause more severe side effects on the kidneys and cardiovascular system.

2.2 Female reproductive tissues

One of OT's traditional target is the pregnant uterus. In rats, the OT gene was found to be expressed in the rat uterine epithelium, amnion, and placenta [14, 15] and humans in amnion, chorion, decidua, and placenta [16]. According to this study result, OT gene expression in chorio-decidual issues was found to have increased three- to fourfold around the time of labor onset [16]. Another research finding also demonstrated that rat uterus OT mRNA increased more than 150-fold at term [14].

However, in maternal plasma, the prominent rise of OT before the onset of labor was not detected in most studies. Besides, the transcriptional level and transcripts of the OT gene are different across organs. Chibbar et.al [16] found that transcriptional levels are highest in the decidua, less in the chorion, and lowest in the placenta. The transcript size in amnion and chorion is larger than the transcript size in the decidua.

There is a popular belief that OT synthesis in gestation is a paracrine system [17]. The known issues include the fetal membranes amnion, chorion and placenta, and the maternal decidua. The location of OT synthesis is parallel with the place where OT gene expression takes place. These OT synthesized by these issues may be the source of OT in amniotic fluid. Possibly, the OT secreted in the form of paracrine is the main source of OT binding with myometrium OTR. This paracrine system was also found in rabbits and bovine [18, 19]. In the pregnant cow, during the whole pregnancy, OT mRNA levels were very low in uterine tissues and appeared to be upregulated at term. Moreover, OT was also found to be synthesized in the corpus luteum. Particularly, after the onset of labor, both OT gene expression and OT peptide are at significant levels in the corpus luteum [18].

Due to the upregulation of OT receptor gene transcription levels and a dramatic rise in OT receptor concentrations in uterine myometrium, uterine sensitivity to OT overtly increases in late pregnancy [14]. The phenomenon is demonstrated both in rat and in human species [15, 20]. It is worthy of noting that OT receptor mRNA expresses highest in the myometrium, low in decidua and chorion, and not detected in the placenta [20], which is in line with the OT gene transcriptional characteristics. Besides, the concentration of oxytocin receptors in the myometrium reaches maximum levels in early labor but in the decidua, the concentration is at peak (nearly five-fold) at parturition [21, 22]. The high concentration of OT receptors in myometrium is relevant to uterine contractility. After parturition, the concentrations of OT receptors decline at a rapid pace. In rats, the uterine OT receptor mRNA levels decreased more than seven-fold within 24 h [23]. The decrease of the OT receptors may be associated with avoiding unnecessary uterus contractility during lactation when maternal OT levels are raised.

Steroid hormones have been proved to be important mediators of OT secretion and OTR gene expression. In 1993, Broad et al. [24] demonstrated that pregnant sheep exposed to progesterone had more OT mRNA in the paraventricular and supraoptic nuclei of the hypothalamus, while those exposed to estrogen didn't show significant growth in the supraoptic nuclei. However, testosterone enhancement during pregnancy brought about decreased oxytocin mRNA expression in the paraventricular nuclei of pregnant rats [25]. Estrogen and testosterone may play an opposite role in the central OT system. While in the peripheral system, estrogens were found to be a strong inductive agent of uterine OT gene expression in the rat uterine, which is seven-fold stronger than progesterone administration [23].

Other hormones also affect the OT. Prostaglandin (PG), essential for parturition, is one of the mediator hormones. Apart from inducing contractions, oxytocin also stimulates prostaglandin synthesis through receptors in the decidua [26]. OT can stimulate the synthesis of PG in the decidua, not in the myometrium *in vitro* [21]. Prostaglandins themselves continue to further uterine contractions, soften the cervix, induce gap-junctions, and intensify the myometrium's sensitivity for oxytocin. At the end of the first stage of labor, the membranes usually rupture leading to a further increase in prostaglandin synthesis, so that once the mechanism is started, it can no longer be interrupted. And OT is a potent stimulator of prostaglandin E_2 synthesis of rabbit amnion cells [27]. According to the study of Gross et.al [28], mice with cyclooxygenase-1 (COX-1), required for the major synthesis of prostaglandin $F_{2\alpha}$ ($PGF_{2\alpha}$), deficiency demonstrated impaired luteolysis, as proved by high serum progesterone concentration and ovarian histology in late pregnancy, as well as delayed induction of uterine oxytocin receptors. Surprisingly, mice deficient in both OT and COX-1 continued to start labor at a normal time. The possible reason for the experiment phenomenon is the opposite effect on the determination of the onset of murine labor-elevated $PGF_{2\alpha}$ production may overcome the luteotrophic action of oxytocin in late gestation. Besides, there may be a crosstalk between OTR and PG receptor [29], because the OTR antagonists not only inhibit OTR but also PG receptors. In summary, OT and its receptors may be regulated by many other hormones, so the interaction between them cannot be ignored in future studies.

3. Oxytocin and behavioral effects

3.1 Maternal behavior

3.1.1 Animal studies

Oxytocin and oxytocin receptors are essential for maternal studies [17, 30, 31]. In oxytocin receptor knockout mice, $Oxtr^{-/-}$ and $Oxtr^{FB/FB}$ mice show largely normal maternal behavior. But it is worth mention that with external disturbance ruled out, $Oxtr^{FB/FB}$ female mice's pups mortality increases compared to wildtype females'. And the possible reasons for the higher mortality are unclear [32]. Interestingly, during maternal retrieval behaviors, there is lateralization in oxytocin receptor expression in the female auditory cortex: more oxytocin receptors are expressed in the left auditory cortex compared to the right auditory cortex in mothers [33].

Most scientific studies suggest that oxytocin is critical to the onset and maintenance of maternal behavior [34]. However, recent research finding of oxytocin receptor gene knockout mice indicates that oxytocin can lower the threshold for the initiation of maternal behavior, however, once the program is started, oxytocin is not crucial to its maintenance [35].

The most recognized understanding of the modification mechanism is the OT-dopamine system: OT circuits interact closely with dopaminergic circuits to mediate maternal behavior. In one research, direct infusion of oxytocin into the ventral tegmental area has been proved to increase the dopamine signal in the nucleus accumbens. Besides, compared with low pup licking/grooming (LG) mothers, high LG mothers show a greater rise in dopamine signal during pup LG behavior, and this alteration diminished with infusions of an oxytocin receptor antagonist directly into the VTA [36]. Studies on OT-related maternal function mechanisms need to expand.

3.1.2 Human studies

Animal research has demonstrated that maternal care behavior pattern varies as the alternation of peripheral OT level across species including sheep [30], monkeys, and rats [31]. Now, many important advances have been extended from animal models to humans, illustrating the role of OT in human mothering behavior. Research in this area has revealed that many factors could result in the individual differences of OT secretion and OT-related functions in women.

Mother-infant attachment is the first important factor. In a control experiment [37], fifty mothers and their 7-month-old infants were divided into two pattern groups: maternal gaze group and maternal gaze toward and gaze shifts away from the infant group, mother's oxytocin response shows a positive correlation with duration of time gaze on her infant and a negative correlation with the frequency of gaze shift from infants. Breastfeeding is another crucial part of mother-infant attachment. There is a research finding that indicates breastfeeding mothers show higher maternal sensitivity when listening to their infants crying compared to formula-feeding in the early postpartum [38]. And other academic study results are consistent with the understanding that mother-infant interaction enhances maternal oxytocin response [39]. Moreover, early caregiving experiences also influence the OT system. Women's levels of CSF OT are positively correlated with the severity and duration of abuse and neglect to which they were exposed in childhood [40]. In females without harsh parenting experiences, the mother's handgrip force (which may be related to sensitive caregiving behavior) decreases in response to infant crying after they intake intranasal oxytocin [41].

Studies also have examined OT-related maternal brain responses. Strathearn et al. discovered that dopamine-associated reward regions, as well as the hypothalamic OT regions, were activated when mothers with secure attachment viewed their infants smiling or crying images [42]. Similar results were reported by Atzil et al. who demonstrated that mothers who displayed synchronous forms of mothering showed activation of the nucleus accumbens, a key reward region while viewing video clips of their infants. Notably, activations in these brain regions were correlated with the peripheral measures of OT in these mothers.

3.2 Mating

OT in human reproduction is involved in both central and peripheral levels. During orgasm, OT acts on the contractions of male and female internal reproductive organs. To the male, OT receptors are linked with semen emission [1], while as to the female, OT receptors within the uterus contribute to uterine contractions. Previous scientific research on the role of OT in human reproduction is mainly concentrated on the periphery. Many studies have proved a prominent increase in plasma OT levels during sexual arousal and immediately the following orgasm in both men and women [43, 44]. However, with the development of neuroimaging techniques, like functional magnetic resonance imaging studies (fMRI) and positron emission tomography (PET), the focus mostly transfers into OT's central effects. To date, many brain areas such as the anterior lobe of the cerebellar vermis and deep cerebellar nuclei respond actively during orgasm [45].

3.2.1 Central OT

For its convivence and intuition, fMRI scanning and PET have become essential tools for research into how central systems regulate human reproduction. As important sexually dimorphic brain regions, the thalamus and hypothalamus play a crucial role in sexual arousal and sexual behavior [46]. During orgasm, women's brain areas included the hypothalamic paraventricular nucleus (PVN)-a major site of OT production and secretion and the periaqueductal gray which receives projections from the PVN show significant activation. Many other brain regions also show activation in mating, such as the medial amygdala, anterior cingulate, nucleus tractus solitarii (NTS), and cerebellar (the anterior lobe of the cerebellar vermis and deep cerebellar nuclei) [45, 46]. However, the association between the activatory regions and the OT system still requires further elucidation.

There is an obvious gender difference in sexual behavior, especially in mating. According to an fMRI study using 20 female and 20 male healthy subjects, when viewing erotic film excerpts, male subjects experience greater sexual arousal (SA).

By analyzing fMRI data, compared with female subjects, male subjects show greater hypothalamic activation, Karama et al. [46] speculate the gender difference may be correlated with activation of the hypothalamus- a brain region that plays an important role in sexual behavior. Other studies involving male subjects also found similar activation of this brain area during erotic visual stimulation [47, 48]. Interestingly, the hypothalamus supraoptic nucleus (SON) and PVN are the main sites of OT gene expression. Besides, only the periaqueductal gray in man where OT was released into prominently activated during orgasm [45].

In summary, there may be some connection between OT and sexual behavior, but the specific mechanism is unclear. Future studies may pay more attention to link brain activation with behavioral effects to figure out the function of central OT in human sexuality. It's worth noting that, although females' hypothalamus activation is interior to males', peripheral OT in both genders shows similarities during sexual arousal.

3.2.2 Peripheral OT

Researchers have attempted to link peripheral OT with reproductive tissues. According to the above, OT receptors within epithelial cells of the epididymis facilitate contractions during ejaculation, contributing to semen emission. These receptors may mediate sperm production as well. In the female, OT receptors exist in the uterus, appearing in higher concentrations during labor. Besides, during the female orgasm, contractions also occur for the activation of OT receptors in the non-pregnant uterus [49]. The role of these contractions is popularly accepted as facilitating sperm transport (often referred to as the "upsuck hypothesis"). A study of 50 women conducted by Wildt et al. [50] supported this hypothesis. Following intravenous OT injection during the follicular stage, a larger number of radiolabeled particles reached the oviduct that contained the dominant follicle, as well as the elevated amplitude of uterine contractions. It is obvious that OT is concerned with human uterine contractions; however, the purpose of these contractions during mating is not clear. It may be responsible for an arousal state in both sexes with exogenous OT exposure.

4. Clinical use of oxytocin

4.1 Autism spectrum disorders

OT has been put into clinical use concerning autism spectrum disorders (ASD). It is important to establish the appropriate dosage that should be given to humans. In a randomized placebo-controlled double-blind crossover trial which is aimed to inquire into OT's dose-dependent effects of a single oxytocin administration in autism, 17 male adults with ASD received 8 international units (IU) oxytocin, 24 IU or placebo before they proceeded four social-cognitive tasks and evaluate the effect of treatment by the measure of overt emotion salience [51]. The research finding suggests that just a low dose of oxytocin can modulate overt emotion salience.

OT's treatment effect works by enhancing brain activity. Under social stimulation, OT selectively improves the brain activity of key areas associated with attention and emotion regulation like the amygdala, hippocampus, mid-orbitofrontal cortex, and insula region [52]. And in another clinical trial, inducing oxytocin can restore brain activity of the medial prefrontal cortex [53].

4.2 Labor induction

OT is a highly efficient and safe agent for the induction the labor and has considerable therapeutic uses. Hofbauer, who first used oxytocin to induce labor, said, "with its power of producing regular, rhythmical and forcible uterine contractions, should be regarded as a most beneficent and valuable agent, which, however, should always be employed with the care of its limitations and dangers." Large-dose OT used in labor induction led to minimal, but not trivial, antidiuretic, and vascular activity [54], which may be associated with the vasopressin and prostaglandin. OT should be used in the lowest possible doses which can induce an effective clinical response.

Patients' resistance to induction or augmentation of labor caused by long-time use of OT in labor induction is not uncommon in the clinical. Daniel-Speigel et al. addressed this issue in a prospective, randomized trial of 104 women who received oxytocin via a low-dose protocol for labor induction. One group of women received intravenous oxytocin until 5-cm dilation, at which time it was discontinued, whereas the other group was continued on the dose of oxytocin that they were receiving at 5-cm dilation. They failed to show any significant difference between groups in the time interval from induction to the active phase, length of the active phase, or length of the second stage of labor. They concluded that continuing oxytocin infusion after the onset of active labor did not seem to have any benefit on the course of labor. In fact, women who received continuous oxytocin infusion throughout their labor course experienced greater rates of uterine hyperstimulation and underwent more cesarean sections. In our practice, we have found that if during induction of labor a high dose of oxytocin has been reached and maintained for a prolonged period and membranes are intact, it is sometimes beneficial to stop the infusion, let the patient rest for several hours, and then begin again. More uterine contractions were induced with each mU of oxytocin infused via pulsatile administration in comparison to using continuous infusion [55]. Different methods of OT infusion may result in discrepancies in labor induction. In patients with prelabor rupture of membranes, a Foley catheter with OT does not shorten the time to delivery compared with OT alone but may contribute to the increase in the chance of intraamniotic infection [56]. Pulsatile administration can prominently reduce the dose of OT required to induce labor [55].

According to the known OT physiological effects, highly specific OT antagonists may be of great therapeutic value for the prevention of preterm labor [57, 58]. To date, many OT antagonists have been developed, the relatively efficient of which is a drug called Retosiban. Retosiban is above 15 times more potent than atosiban which is a marketed intravenous OT antagonist at the human oxytocin receptor, as evidenced by effective inhibition of uterus contractions by intravenous and by oral administration in rats [59]. Moreover, antagonists of OT can also be used to treat dysmenorrhea by relaxing the uterine myometrium [60].

5. Summary

The link between OT oxytocin and pregnancy is explored in three aspects: physiology, ethology, and clinical application. A conclusion can be drawn from the above: the link between OT and pregnancy appears to be strong, both in the first and second trimesters, especially in the third trimester. Although most of the OT mechanisms and effects are known, there are still some suspects, for example, what's the function of the contraction caused by OT during orgasm. Additionally, whether the OT synthesized in different parts can be transported to other parts to do their job? And if so, how do they communicate? Apart from the classical effect, in recent years, the role of oxytocin in behavior has received increasing attention. OT disorder is related to behavioral disorders like childhood cognitive impairment, ASD, and maternal postpartum depression [61], but as far as the scientific research is concerned, the mechanism of this phenomenon is not very specific. And as such, to explain this phenomenon, more efforts are needed in the future. Last but not least, although OT has rare side effects on the human body, it is still worth discussing how to use OT safely and efficiently in clinical practice. In conclusion, OT is essential for pregnancy, and more detailed function mechanism should be explored in future research.

Acknowledgements

This work was supported by National Natural Science Foundation of China (81971405, 81673217), Major Natural Science Research Projects of Jiangsu University (20KJA330001), Medical Research Project of Jiangsu Health Commission (Z2019010), and the Priority Academic Program for the Development of Jiangsu Higher Education Institutions (Public Health and Preventive Medicine).

Author details

Haiwen Yu[1,2], Yuting Cheng[1,2], Yiwen Lu[1,2], Wei Wu[1,2]* and Qiuqin Tang[3]*

1 State Key Laboratory of Reproductive Medicine, Institute of Toxicology, Nanjing Medical University, Nanjing, China

2 Key Laboratory of Modern Toxicology of Ministry of Education, School of Public Health, Nanjing Medical University, Nanjing, China

3 Department of Obstetrics, Women's Hospital of Nanjing Medical University, Nanjing Maternity and Child Health Care Hospital, Nanjing, China

*Address all correspondence to: wwu@njmu.edu.cn and t19871004@sina.com

References

[1] Gimpl G, Fahrenholz F. The oxytocin receptor system: structure, function, and regulation. Physiol Rev. 2001;81(2): 629-83.

[2] Telgmann R, Bathgate RAD, Jaeger S, Tillmann G, Ivell R. Transcriptional regulation of the bovine oxytocin receptor gene. Biol Reprod. 2003;68(3): 1015-26.

[3] Frayne J, Nicholson HD. Localization of oxytocin receptors in the human and macaque monkey male reproductive tracts: evidence for a physiological role of oxytocin in the male. Mol Hum Reprod. 1998;4(6):527-32.

[4] Bathgate RA, Sernia C. Characterization and localization of oxytocin receptors in the rat testis. J Endocrinol. 1994;141(2):343-52.

[5] Parry LJ, Bathgate RA. Mesotocin receptor gene and protein expression in the prostate gland, but not testis, of the tammar wallaby, *Macropus eugenii*. Biol Reprod. 1998;59(5):1101-7.

[6] Pickering BT, Birkett SD, Guldenaar SE, Nicholson HD, Worley RT, Yavachev L. Oxytocin in the testis: what, where, and why? Ann N Y Acad Sci. 1989;564:198-209.

[7] Anjum S, Anuradha A, Krishna A. A possible direct action of oxytocin on spermatogenesis and steroidogenesis in pre-pubertal mouse. Andrologia. 2018;e12958.

[8] Harris GC, Nicholson HD. Characterisation of the biological effects of neurohypophysial peptides on seminiferous tubules. J Endocrinol. 1998;156(1):35-42.

[9] Frayne J, Townsend D, Nicholson HD. Effects of oxytocin on sperm transport in the pubertal rat. J Reprod Fertil. 1996;107(2):299-306.

[10] Gerendai I, Csernus V. Effect of intratesticular administration of oxytocin on testicular steroidogenesis in immature rats. Andrologia. 1995;27(5):291-7.

[11] Sharpe RM, Cooper I. Comparison of the effects on purified Leydig cells of four hormones (oxytocin, vasopressin, opiates and LHRH) with suggested paracrine roles in the testis. J Endocrinol. 1987;113(1):89-96.

[12] Song Z, Albers HE. Cross-talk among oxytocin and arginine-vasopressin receptors: Relevance for basic and clinical studies of the brain and periphery. Front Neuroendocrinol. 2018;51:14-24.

[13] Gupta J, Russell R, Wayman C, Hurley D, Jackson V. Oxytocin-induced contractions within rat and rabbit ejaculatory tissues are mediated by vasopressin V1A receptors and not oxytocin receptors. Br J Pharmacol. 2008;155(1):118-26.

[14] Lefebvre DL, Giaid A, Bennett H, Larivière R, Zingg HH. Oxytocin gene expression in rat uterus. Science. 1992;256(5063):1553-5.

[15] Lefebvre DL, Lariviere R, Zingg HH. Rat amnion: a novel site of oxytocin production. Biol Reprod. 1993;48(3):632-9.

[16] Chibbar R, Miller FD, Mitchell BF. Synthesis of oxytocin in amnion, chorion, and decidua may influence the timing of human parturition. J Clin Invest. 1993;91(1):185-92.

[17] Mitchell BF, Fang X, Wong S. Oxytocin: a paracrine hormone in the regulation of parturition? Rev Reprod. 1998;3(2):113-22.

[18] Ivell R, Rust W, Einspanier A, Hartung S, Fields M, Fuchs AR. Oxytocin and oxytocin receptor gene

expression in the reproductive tract of the pregnant cow: rescue of luteal oxytocin production at term. Biol Reprod. 1995;53(3):553-60.

[19] Jeng YJ, Lolait SJ, Soloff MS. Induction of oxytocin receptor gene expression in rabbit amnion cells. Endocrinology. 1998;139(8):3449-55.

[20] Wathes DC, Borwick SC, Timmons PM, Leung ST, Thornton S. Oxytocin receptor expression in human term and preterm gestational tissues prior to and following the onset of labour. J Endocrinol. 1999;161(1):143-51.

[21] Fuchs AR, Fuchs F, Husslein P, Soloff MS, Fernström MJ. Oxytocin receptors and human parturition: a dual role for oxytocin in the initiation of labor. Science. 1982;215(4538):1396-8.

[22] Soloff MS, Fernstrom MA, Periyasamy S, Soloff S, Baldwin S, Wieder M. Regulation of oxytocin receptor concentration in rat uterine explants by estrogen and progesterone. Can J Biochem Cell Biol. 1983;61(7): 625-30.

[23] Zingg HH, Rozen F, Breton C, Larcher A, Neculcea J, Chu K, et al. Gonadal steroid regulation of oxytocin and oxytocin receptor gene expression. Adv Exp Med Biol. 1995;395:395-404.

[24] Broad KD, Kendrick KM, Sirinathsinghji DJ, Keverne EB. Changes in oxytocin immunoreactivity and mRNA expression in the sheep brain during pregnancy, parturition and lactation and in response to oestrogen and progesterone. J Neuroendocrinol. 1993;5(4): 435-44.

[25] Dzirbíková Z, Talarovičová A, Štefánik P, Olexová L, Kršková L. Testosterone enhancement during pregnancy influences social coping and gene expression of oxytocin and vasopressin in the brain of adult rats. Acta Neurobiol Exp (Wars). 2018;78(3):264-70.

[26] Husslein P. [Causes of labor initiation in man: role of oxytocin and prostaglandins]. Z Geburtshilfe Perinatol. 1985;189(3):95-102.

[27] Hinko A, Soloff MS. Characterization of oxytocin receptors in rabbit amnion involved in the production of prostaglandin E2. Endocrinology. 1992;130(6):3547-53.

[28] Gross GA, Imamura T, Luedke C, Vogt SK, Olson LM, Nelson DM, et al. Opposing actions of prostaglandins and oxytocin determine the onset of murine labor. Proc Natl Acad Sci USA. 1998;95(20):11875-9.

[29] Kim SH, Riaposova L, Ahmed H, Pohl O, Chollet A, Gotteland J-P, et al. Oxytocin Receptor Antagonists, Atosiban and Nolasiban, Inhibit Prostaglandin F-induced Contractions and Inflammatory Responses in Human Myometrium. Sci Rep. 2019;9(1):5792.

[30] Kendrick KM, Keverne EB, Baldwin BA. Intracerebroventricular oxytocin stimulates maternal behaviour in the sheep. Neuroendocrinology. 1987;46(1):56-61.

[31] Pedersen CA, Prange AJ. Induction of maternal behavior in virgin rats after intracerebroventricular administration of oxytocin. Proc Natl Acad Sci USA. 1979;76(12):6661-5.

[32] Macbeth AH, Stepp JE, Lee HJ, Young WS, 3rd, Caldwell HK. Normal maternal behavior, but increased pup mortality, in conditional oxytocin receptor knockout females. Behav Neurosci. 2010;124(5):677-85.

[33] Marlin BJ, Mitre M, D'Amour J A, Chao MV, Froemke RC. Oxytocin enables maternal behaviour by balancing cortical inhibition. Nature. 2015;520(7548):499-504.

[34] Kim S, Soeken TA, Cromer SJ, Martinez SR, Hardy LR, Strathearn L. Oxytocin and postpartum depression: delivering on what's known and what's not. Brain Res. 2014;1580:219-32.

[35] Rich ME, deCardenas EJ, Lee HJ, Caldwell HK. Impairments in the initiation of maternal behavior in oxytocin receptor knockout mice. PLoS One. 2014;9(6):e98839.

[36] Shahrokh DK, Zhang TY, Diorio J, Gratton A, Meaney MJ. Oxytocin-dopamine interactions mediate variations in maternal behavior in the rat. Endocrinology. 2010;151(5):2276-86.

[37] Kim S, Fonagy P, Koos O, Dorsett K, Strathearn L. Maternal oxytocin response predicts mother-to-infant gaze. Brain Res. 2014;1580:133-42.

[38] Kim P, Feldman R, Mayes LC, Eicher V, Thompson N, Leckman JF, et al. Breastfeeding, brain activation to own infant cry, and maternal sensitivity. J Child Psychol Psychiatry. 2011;52(8): 907-15.

[39] Feldman R, Gordon I, Schneiderman I, Weisman O, Zagoory-Sharon O. Natural variations in maternal and paternal care are associated with systematic changes in oxytocin following parent-infant contact. Psychoneuroendocrinology. 2010;35(8):1133-41.

[40] Heim C, Young LJ, Newport DJ, Mletzko T, Miller AH, Nemeroff CB. Lower CSF oxytocin concentrations in women with a history of childhood abuse. Mol Psychiatry. 2009;14(10): 954-8.

[41] Bakermans-Kranenburg MJ, van Ijzendoorn MH, Riem MM, Tops M, Alink LR. Oxytocin decreases handgrip force in reaction to infant crying in females without harsh parenting experiences. Soc Cogn Affect Neurosci. 2012;7(8):951-7.

[42] Strathearn L, Fonagy P, Amico J, Montague PR. Adult attachment predicts maternal brain and oxytocin response to infant cues. Neuropsychopharmacology. 2009;34(13):2655-66.

[43] Murphy MR, Checkley SA, Seckl JR, Lightman SL. Naloxone inhibits oxytocin release at orgasm in man. J Clin Endocrinol Metab. 1990;71(4): 1056-8.

[44] Salonia A, Nappi RE, Pontillo M, Daverio R, Smeraldi A, Briganti A, et al. Menstrual cycle-related changes in plasma oxytocin are relevant to normal sexual function in healthy women. Horm Behav. 2005;47(2):164-9.

[45] Georgiadis JR, Reinders AA, Paans AM, Renken R, Kortekaas R. Men versus women on sexual brain function: prominent differences during tactile genital stimulation, but not during orgasm. Hum Brain Mapp. 2009;30(10): 3089-101.

[46] Karama S, Lecours AR, Leroux JM, Bourgouin P, Beaudoin G, Joubert S, et al. Areas of brain activation in males and females during viewing of erotic film excerpts. Hum Brain Mapp. 2002;16(1):1-13.

[47] Brunetti M, Babiloni C, Ferretti A, Del Gratta C, Merla A, Olivetti Belardinelli M, et al. Hypothalamus, sexual arousal and psychosexual identity in human males: a functional magnetic resonance imaging study. Eur J Neurosci. 2008;27(11):2922-7.

[48] Ferretti A, Caulo M, Del Gratta C, Di Matteo R, Merla A, Montorsi F, et al. Dynamics of male sexual arousal: distinct components of brain activation revealed by fMRI. Neuroimage. 2005;26(4):1086-96.

[49] Meston CM, Levin RJ, Sipski ML, Hull EM, Heiman JR. Women's orgasm. Annu Rev Sex Res. 2004;15:173-257.

[50] Wildt L, Kissler S, Licht P, Becker W. Sperm transport in the human female genital tract and its modulation by oxytocin as assessed by hysterosalpingoscintigraphy, hysterotonography, electrohystero graphy and Doppler sonography. Hum Reprod Update. 1998;4(5):655-66.

[51] Quintana DS, Westlye LT, Hope S, Naerland T, Elvsashagen T, Dorum E, et al. Dose-dependent social-cognitive effects of intranasal oxytocin delivered with novel Breath Powered device in adults with autism spectrum disorder: a randomized placebo-controlled double-blind crossover trial. Transl Psychiatry. 2017;7(5):e1136.

[52] Andari E, Richard N, Leboyer M, Sirigu A. Adaptive coding of the value of social cues with oxytocin, an fMRI study in autism spectrum disorder. Cortex. 2016;76:79-88.

[53] Watanabe T, Abe O, Kuwabara H, Yahata N, Takano Y, Iwashiro N, et al. Mitigation of sociocommunicational deficits of autism through oxytocin-induced recovery of medial prefrontal activity: a randomized trial. JAMA Psychiatry. 2014;71(2):166-75.

[54] Shyken JM, Petrie RH. Oxytocin to induce labor. Clin Obstet Gynecol. 1995;38(2):232-45.

[55] Randolph GW, Fuchs AR. Pulsatile administration enhances the effect and reduces the dose of oxytocin required for induction of labor. Am J Perinatol. 1989;6(2):159-66.

[56] Mackeen AD, Durie DE, Lin M, Huls CK, Qureshey E, Paglia MJ, et al. Foley Plus Oxytocin Compared With Oxytocin for Induction After Membrane Rupture: A Randomized Controlled Trial. Obstet Gynecol. 2018;131(1):4-11.

[57] Williams PD, Bock MG, Tung RD, Garsky VM, Perlow DS, Erb JM, et al. Development of a novel class of cyclic hexapeptide oxytocin antagonists based on a natural product. J Med Chem. 1992;35(21):3905-18.

[58] Evans BE, Leighton JL, Rittle KE, Gilbert KF, Lundell GF, Gould NP, et al. Orally active, nonpeptide oxytocin antagonists. J Med Chem. 1992;35(21): 3919-27.

[59] Borthwick AD, Liddle J. The design of orally bioavailable 2, 5-diketopiperazine oxytocin antagonists: from concept to clinical candidate for premature labor. Med Res Rev. 2011;31(4):576-604.

[60] Akerlund M. Targeting the oxytocin receptor to relax the myometrium. Expert Opin Ther Targets. 2006;10(3): 423-7.

[61] Freedman D, Brown AS, Shen L, Schaefer CA. Perinatal oxytocin increases the risk of offspring bipolar disorder and childhood cognitive impairment. J Affect Disord. 2015;173:65-72.

Chapter 2

Molecular Aspects and Structure Activity Relationship of Oxytocin Agonists and Antagonist's Role in Health

Veera C.S.R. Chittepu, Poonam Kalhotra, Tzayhri Gallardo Velazquez and Guillermo Osorio Revilla

Abstract

Oxytocin (OT) and Oxytocin receptor signaling mechanism had emerged as a pathway for treatment of metabolic disorders like obesity, and diabetes. Both agonists and antagonists activity of the oxytocin receptor has beneficial aspects. This chapter will outline the receptor agonists and antagonist's activity as a function of the features: hydrophobic regions, activity shapes, and positive and negative electrostatics. Also, their phenotype characteristics in various diseases like diabetes, obesity, cardiovascular and immune related diseases will be outlined. Finally, therapeutic development strategies for using various nanomaterials, and other biomaterials, as well as those in present use will be discussed.

Keywords: oxytocin, agonists and antagonists, drug delivery, nanomaterials, biomaterials, diabetes, obesity, regenerative medicine

1. Introduction

Oxytocin (OT) was the first hormone to have its composition determined and was synthesized in a biologically active manner [1]. OT is a major neuropeptide, and its roles involve control of neuroendocrine reflexes [2], the development of particular social and bonding habits [3], and the reproductive and maternal functions [4]. Cyclic nonapeptide OT and its structurally related peptides facilitate reproduction in many vertebrates.

In earlier years, OT was believed to be restricted to stimulate uterine contractions during childbirth [5] and milking (lactation) but the fact that OT is found in both men and women in the brain and plasma indicates there are other significant roles.

Most of the OT like peptides are nonapeptides and have a disulfide bridge between cysteine residues 1 and 6. The residue Lysine at position 3 and arginine or lysine at position 8 are responsible for biological activity of oxytocin peptide, that is, to activate oxytocin receptor [1]. Generally, the nonapeptides are classified as vasopressins and OT families, and are based on the presence of basic amino acid at position 8 and neutral amino acids. **Figure 1** shows the phylogenetic tree corresponding to oxytocin like peptides, retrieved from Uniprot webpage [6].

The oxytocin gene is located on chromosome 3p25 and comprises 3 introns and 4 exons and belongs to the G protein-coupled receptor (GPCR) superfamily. Oxytocin binds to receptors that activate intracellular signaling pathways, triggering the activation of proteins. **Figure 2** was developed by the authors to show in a schematic way, the oxytocin-oxytocin receptor (OT-OTR) signaling pathway in the body. Upon binding OT to OTR, Gq/phospholipase C (PLC)/inositol

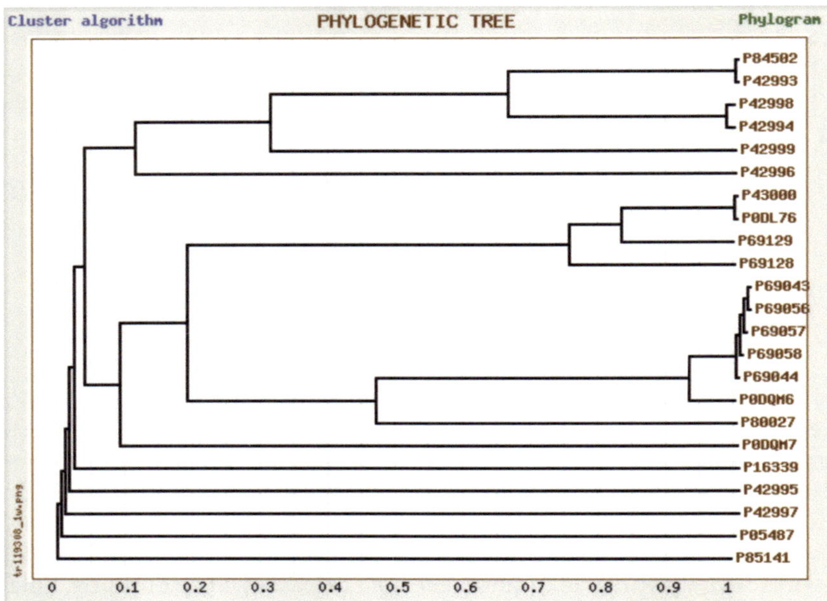

Figure 1.
Phylogenetic tree of oxytocin like peptides. Oxytocin like peptides are denoted using their Uniprot ID (Uniprot webpage [6]).

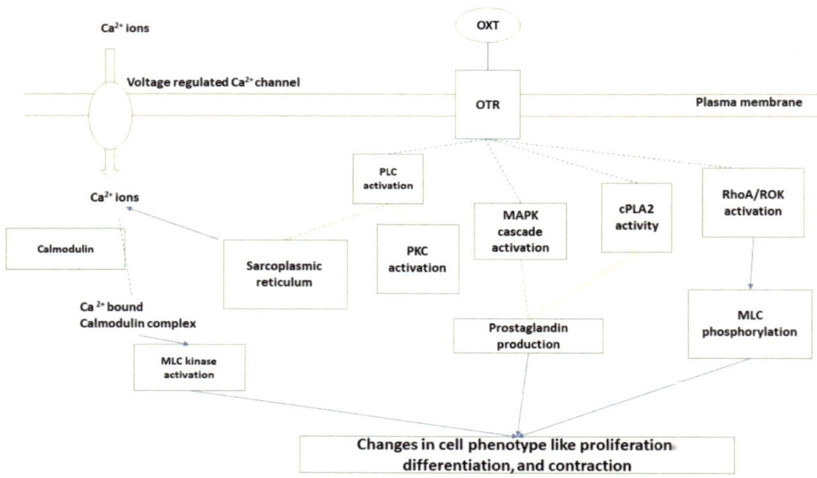

Figure 2.
Molecular features of oxytocin receptor modulators calculated using forge tool. Oxytocin receptor linked signaling pathways resulting in cell phenotype. OT: Oxytocin, OTR: Oxytocin receptor, PLC: Phospholipase, PIP2: Phosphatidylinositol 4,5-bisphosphate, InsP3: Inositol 1,4,5- triphosphate, DAG: Diacylglycerol, PKC: Protein kinases type C, MLC: Myosin light-chain, MAPK: Mitogen-activated protein kinase, cPLA2: Cytosolic phospholipase A2, ROK: RhoA associated protein kinase.

1,4,5-triphosphate (InsP3) pathway dominates the phosphatidylinositol 4,5-bisphosphate (PIP2) hydrolysis and this results in InsP3 and diacylglycerol (DAG) (DAG). InsP3 releases Ca^{2+} ions from the intracellular sarcoplasmic reticulum stores, but the DAG further activates protein kinases which phosphorylate other proteins. Mammary epithelial cells and milk ejection is caused by Ca^{2+} ions. Activation of MAPK cascade is triggered by OTR and PKC resulting in increased expression of cPLA2 activity, which eventually results in development of prostaglandins. The profusion of prostaglandins development often causes muscle contractions. OTR activation elicits phosphorylation of calcineurin. All these signaling pathways result in many cellular effects such as cell formation, cell differentiation, and motility.

Transmembrane domains 3,4, and 6 of oxytocin receptor forms the docking site to oxytocin peptide cyclic part, and other c terminal domain of oxytocin interacts closely with domain 2 and domain 3 in the extracellular space of the oxytocin receptor. The key OTR residues R34, F103, D85, F284, and Y209, play a role in selectivity of oxytocin peptide. Based on the activity of oxytocin receptor, the oxytocin analogues were classified as agonists and antagonists.

2. OTR agonists and antagonists

Receptor binding and functional studies were generally used to identify oxytocin receptor agonists and antagonist activity. There are more than thousand compounds in literature as OTR agonists and antagonists, and this section was focused to demonstrate the applicability of molecular shape features as tool to develop agonists and antagonists. For this reason, peptide agonist and antagonist molecular shapes features are compared with oxytocin.

Substitution of hydoxyl group at position 1 and threonine at position 4 of original oxytocin peptide (peptide 1, **Figure 3**) revealed highest affinity to oxytocin receptor (OTR), with value of Ki 0.31 nM and served as oxytocin agonist and as a possible treatment of autism [7], and for the treatment of postpartum hemorrhage [8].

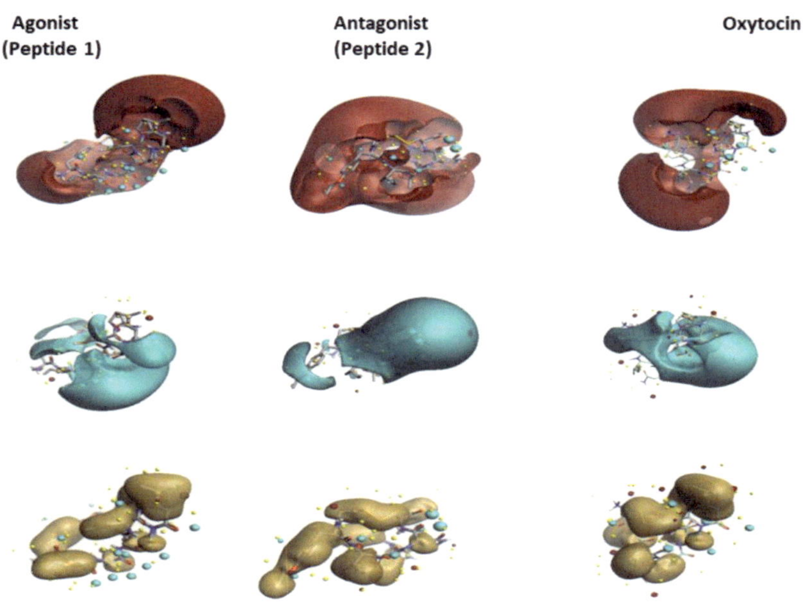

Figure 3.
Molecular features of oxytocin receptor modulators calculated using forge tool.

Peptide atosiban (peptide 2, **Figure 3**) revealed affinity to oxytocin receptor with a value of Ki 76 nM, and it is used in clinical as oxytocin antagonist [9]. Newly developed Cresset XED force field provided by software Forge [10] was utilized to understand the key features of oxytocin, agonist and antagonist of oxytocin receptor.

Figure 3 was developed by the authors using Forge tool for oxytocin, agonist and antagonist of OTR, and features were visualized using Forge visualization software to show the comparison of features: red color (positive electrostatics), blue color (negative electrostatics), and gold color (hydrophobic shapes).

The molecular features shown in **Figure 3** are the result of activities and clearly reveal agonist and antagonist function on the oxytocin receptor. Visual examination either manually or using imaging algorithms of all the fields, reveals the presence of positive electrostatic feature in definite coordinates, and size and shape are responsible for agonist and antagonist activity of OTR. Increased electronegative regions favor agonist activity, and similarly, hydrophobic shape features are distinct for agonist and antagonist activity of OTR. The features mentioned in this study, indeed can be utilized by various investigators to discover, develop, and optimize agonist and antagonists of OTR. It is well possible to screen various libraries and chose the molecules of interest.

3. Phenotype characteristics in various diseases

Oxytocin receptor agonists and antagonists has potential benefits in health care, especially in treating diabetes, obesity, cardiovascular, and immune related disorders. It is well known that diabetes is considered one of the major causes of mortality and a metabolic disorder. Incidence of diabetes mellitus will increases over coming decades and is generally considered that affect many organs [11]. Many researchers has demonstrated beneficial effect of oxytocin, as endogenous factor, with significant changes in insulin sensitivity [12], lipidomic [13], and glucose metabolism [14]. Oxytocin stimulates glucose uptake [14, 15], and glucagon secretion [16] in pancreatic islets which is directly implicated in improvement and involvement of pathophysiology of diabetes.

Apart from diabetes, another major problem most of countries are concerned about is obesity, both in Mexico and worldwide [17, 18]. Oxytocin is well known for its effects in control of the energy balance [19]. It's well proven that oxytocin administration reduces body weight [20], food intake [21], and glucose tolerance was observed with administration of oxytocin [22]. In addition, oxytocin administration induces a marker of neuronal activation that is known as Fos [23], that is linked to control meal size, regulation of intake of food and indeed bodyweight.

Another class of disease is cardiovascular disease, where 13% of deaths are due to this, specifically due to blood pressure, followed by tobacco, diabetes, and lack of exercise [24]. Cardiovascular diseases involve generally blood vessels or heart [25]. Oxytocin receptor decreases blood pressure [26] and lowers brain natriuretic peptide [27]. Oxytocin was also proven to facilitate the recovery of cardiovascular system (CVS) [28] from injuries [29] and decrease progression of atherosclerosis. Key pathways involved in cardiovascular protection upon treatment with oxytocin act by suppressing the increasing production of cytokines, apoptotic pathways are activated through the involvement of multiple signaling pathways [29].

Oxytocin is also involved in immune related health problem; oxytocin was proven to trigger thymocyte proliferation [30], inducing immune tolerance, which is generally observed in thymus which is a primary tissue responsible for [31]. The nonapeptide oxytocin interacts with neurohypophysial peptide receptors expressed by pre-T cells and induces phosphorylation of focal adhesion kinase [32]. Generally, oxytocin production decreases with age, which is linked to thymic involution. Oxytocin also has antiviral activity and it has been reported its possible used to treat CoVID-19 through DPP-inhibition mechanism of action [33, 34].

4. Nano, micro and macro materials for delivery of agonists and antagonists

Up today, oxytocin receptor agonists and antagonists formulations including nano, micro and macro materials are not available in the market. Existing oxytocin receptor agonists and antagonists possess drawbacks like lack of efficacy, no improvement in neonatal outcomes, low stability, short half-life in-vivo, and low bioavailability.

Many researchers had started to utilize alternative approaches to address mentioned drawbacks, and among these, encapsulations for slow and steady oxytocin release are under investigation. Most of them are polymeric carriers, and liposome-based technologies.

Among the polymeric carriers for oxytocin, solvent displacement method was utilized to synthesize poloxamer hydrogel scaffold, to encapsulate oxytocin in hydrogel graft constituted of poly(d, l-lactide-co-glycolide) (PLGA), β-tricalcium phosphate, and hydroxyapatite (CP). This method yielded 89.5% encapsulation efficiency, slowly release encapsulated oxytocin, and finally yielded significant regeneration of bone loss in rat calvaria [35].

Another nanomaterial application was based on Bovine Serum Albumin (BSA) based nanocomposites. It is a twostep process to synthesize nanocomposites, nanoprecipitation followed by lyophilization. Transferrin (Tf) and Rabies Virus Glycoprotein (RVG) was conjugated to synthesized oxytocin-BSA nanoparticles for successful delivery of oxytocin across blood brain barrier (BBB). This composite was delivered intranasally, and an improvement in oxytocin bioavailability was observed. Delivery of oxytocin using nanocomposites led to greater pro-social effects in comparison to oxytocin alone within 3 days of intranasal administration. This delivery system definitely benefits social-deficit disorders and indeed enhance the brain delivery peptides [36].

Another important nanocarrier utilized in successful delivery oxytocin receptor agonists and antagonists is liposomal drug delivery systems. In specific, antibody-based liposomes were applied where PEGylated liposomes were conjugated with atosiban (ATO-Lipo, OTR antagonist) or anti-OTR monoclonal antibodies (OTR-Lipo) using the technology of dried lipid film hydration. This method increased intracellular internalization, and revealed that the cellular uptake is dependent on caveolin-mediated mechanisms, with no cellular toxicity observed. Antibody-conjugated liposomes gave way to improved treatment for obstetric complications [37].

5. Future perspectives

Since the therapeutic effects of agonists and antagonists are growing, more studies will be needed to protect them against biodegradation, to increase intestinal absorption particularly with use of technologies, such as enhancer absorption (cyclodextrines), surfactants, cell penetration peptide, chemistry modifications, nano, micro and macromaterials.

Besides improving drug delivery methods, additional cell-based experiments are required to understand the role of oxytocin such as the use of fluorescent tags

(HaloTag) to monitor new functions for agonists or antagonists, the use of imaging techniques to classify and develop imaging biomarkers is needed to explore the ability of oxytocin receptor agonists or antagonists across tissues, cell-host interactions. In addition, the molecular features described in this study can be used to discover new and novel oxytocin receptor agonists and antagonists.

6. Conclusion

Molecular shape features of oxytocin receptor agonist and antagonist activity as a function of positive and negative electrostatic, and hydrophobic shapes features were developed and detailed. Also, liposome and polymeric based strategies in improving most of the drawbacks associated with oxytocin delivery were discussed. More studies are needed towards the application of diverse nanomaterials to deliver neuropeptides and improve their efficacy. Some of the tools proposed in this chapter can guide the future research in improving the delivery strategies of oxytocin receptor agonists and antagonists.

It has to be remembered that, technologies need to be developed for each route of administration, maintain stability, and steady state release of encapsulated active ingredients.

Acknowledgements

All authors would like to thank for the support provided by Consejo Nacional de Ciencia y Tecnología (CONACYT), Escuela Nacional de Ciencia de Biologicas (ENCB) and Instituto Politecnico Nacional (IPN).\.

Conflict of interest

The authors declare no conflict of interest.

Author details

Veera C.S.R. Chittepu[1], Poonam Kalhotra[2], Tzayhri Gallardo Velazquez[2] and Guillermo Osorio Revilla[1*]

1 Departamento de Ingeniería Bioquímica, Escuela Nacional de Ciencias Biológicas, Instituto Politecnico Nacional, Av. Wilfrido Massieu S/N, Col. Unidad Profesional Adolfo López Mateos, Zacatenco, Ciudad de México, CP, Mexico

2 Departamento de Biofísica, Escuela Nacional de Ciencias Biológicas, Instituto Politécnico Nacional, Prolongación de Carpio y Plan de Ayala S/N, Col. Santo Tomás, Ciudad de México, CP, México

*Address all correspondence to: osorgi@gmail.com

References

[1] Gimpl G, Fahrenholz F (2001) The oxytocin receptor system: Structure, function, and regulation. Physiol Rev. https://doi.org/10.1152/physrev.2001.81.2.629

[2] Bisset GW, Chowdrey HS (1988) CONTROL OF RELEASE OF VASOPRESSIN BY NEUROENDOCRINE REFLEXES. Q J Exp Physiol. https://doi.org/10.1113/expphysiol.1988.sp003223

[3] Lim MM, Young LJ (2006) Neuropeptidergic regulation of affiliative behavior and social bonding in animals. Horm Behav. https://doi.org/10.1016/j.yhbeh.2006.06.028

[4] Burbach JPH, Young LJ, Russell JA (2006) Oxytocin: Synthesis, secretion, and reproductive functions. Knobil Neill's Physiol Reprod. https://doi.org/10.1016/B978-012515400-0/50063-4

[5] Khajehei M (2017) Labour and beyond: The roles of synthetic and endogenous oxytocin in transition to motherhood. Br J Midwifery. https://doi.org/10.12968/bjom.2017.25.4.230

[6] Bateman A, Martin MJ, O'Donovan C, et al (2017) UniProt: The universal protein knowledgebase. Nucleic Acids Res. https://doi.org/10.1093/nar/gkw1099

[7] Hollander E, Bartz J, Chaplin W, Phillips A, Sumner J, Soorya L, Anagnostou E, Wasserman S (2007) Oxytocin Increases Retention of Social Cognition in Autism. Biol Psychiatry. https://doi.org/10.1016/j.biopsych.2006.05.030

[8] Su LL, Chong YS, Samuel M (2007) Oxytocin agonists for preventing postpartum haemorrhage. Cochrane Database Syst Rev. https://doi.org/10.1002/14651858.CD005457.pub2

[9] Manning M, Cheng LL, Stoev S, Ching Wo N, Chan WY, Szeto HH, Durroux T, Mouillac B, Barberis C (2005) Design of peptide oxytocin antagonists with strikingly higher affinities and selectivities for the human oxytocin receptor than atosiban. J Pept Sci. https://doi.org/10.1002/psc.667

[10] Kalhotra P, Chittepu V, Osorio-Revilla G, Gallardo-Velázquez T (2018) Structure–Activity Relationship and Molecular Docking of Natural Product Library Reveal Chrysin as a Novel Dipeptidyl Peptidase-4 (DPP-4) Inhibitor: An Integrated In Silico and In Vitro Study. Molecules 23:1368

[11] Dabelea D, Bell RA, D'Agostino RB, et al (2007) Incidence of diabetes in youth in the United States. J Am Med Assoc. https://doi.org/10.1001/jama.297.24.2716

[12] Zhang H, Wu C, Chen Q, Chen X, Xu Z, Wu J, Cai D (2013) Treatment of Obesity and Diabetes Using Oxytocin or Analogs in Patients and Mouse Models. PLoS One. https://doi.org/10.1371/journal.pone.0061477

[13] Elabd SK, Sabry I, Mohasseb M, Algendy A (2014) Oxytocin as a novel therapeutic option for type I diabetes and diabetic osteopathy. Endocr Regul. https://doi.org/10.4149/endo_2014_02_87

[14] Gutkowska J, Jankowski M (2012) Oxytocin Revisited: Its Role in Cardiovascular Regulation. J Neuroendocrinol. https://doi.org/10.1111/j.1365-2826.2011.02235.x

[15] Florian M, Jankowski M, Gutkowska J (2010) Oxytocin increases glucose uptake in neonatal rat cardiomyocytes. Endocrinology. https://doi.org/10.1210/en.2009-0624

[16] Vilhardt H, Krarup T, Holst JJ, Bie P (1986) The mechanism of the effect of

oxytocin on plasma concentrations of glucose, insulin and glucagon in conscious dogs. J Endocrinol. https://doi.org/10.1677/joe.0.1080293

[17] Haua-Navarro K (2016) Overweight and obesity. Gac Med Mex. https://doi.org/10.4324/9781003139157-7

[18] World Health Organization (2011) Fact Sheet Obesity and overweight. World Heal. Organ.

[19] Zhang G, Bai H, Zhang H, Dean C, Wu Q, Li J, Guariglia S, Meng Q, Cai D (2011) Neuropeptide Exocytosis Involving Synaptotagmin-4 and Oxytocin in Hypothalamic Programming of Body Weight and Energy Balance. Neuron. https://doi.org/10.1016/j.neuron.2010.12.036

[20] Blevins JE, Baskin DG (2015) Translational and therapeutic potential of oxytocin as an anti-obesity strategy: Insights from rodents, nonhuman primates and humans. Physiol Behav. https://doi.org/10.1016/j.physbeh.2015.05.023

[21] Ott V, Finlayson G, Lehnert H, Heitmann B, Heinrichs M, Born J, Hallschmid M (2013) Oxytocin reduces reward-driven food intake in humans. Diabetes. https://doi.org/10.2337/db13-0663

[22] Olson BR, Drutarosky MD, Chow MS, Hruby VJ, Stricker EM, Verbalis JG (1991) Oxytocin and an oxytocin agonist administered centrally decrease food intake in rats. Peptides. https://doi.org/10.1016/0196-9781(91)90176-P

[23] Seeley RJ, Yagaloff KA, Fisher SL, Burn P, Thiele TE, Van Dijk G, Baskin DG, Schwartz MW (1997) Melanocortin receptors in leptin effects. Nature. https://doi.org/10.1038/37016

[24] Mendis S, Puska P, Norrving B (2011) Global atlas on cardiovascular disease prevention and control. World Heal. Organ.

[25] Mackay, Judith, Mensah GA (2004) Types of Cardiovascular Diseases. Atlas Hear. Dis. Stroke

[26] Japundzic-Zigon N (2013) Vasopressin and Oxytocin in Control of the Cardiovascular System. Curr Neuropharmacol. https://doi.org/10.2174/1570159x11311020008

[27] Gutkowska J, Jankowski M, Lambert C, Mukaddam-Daher S, Zingg HH, McCann SM (1997) Oxytocin releases atrial natriuretic peptide by combining with oxytocin receptors in the heart. Proc Natl Acad Sci U S A. https://doi.org/10.1073/pnas.94.21.11704

[28] Petersson M (2002) Cardiovascular effects of oxytocin. Prog Brain Res. https://doi.org/10.1016/S0079-6123(02)39024-1

[29] Wang P, Wang SC, Yang H, et al (2019) Therapeutic potential of oxytocin in atherosclerotic cardiovascular disease: Mechanisms and signaling pathways. Front Neurosci. https://doi.org/10.3389/fnins.2019.00454

[30] Geenen V, Legros JJ, Franchimont P, Baudrihaye M, Defresne MP, Boniver J (1986) The neuroendocrine thymus: Coexistence of oxytocin and neurophysin in the human thymus. Science (80-). https://doi.org/10.1126/science.3961493

[31] Nikolich-Žugich J, Slifka MK, Messaoudi I (2004) The many important facets of T-cell repertoire diversity. Nat Rev Immunol. https://doi.org/10.1038/nri1292

[32] Martens H, Kecha O, Charlet-Renard C, Defresne MP, Geenen V (1998) Neurohypophysial peptides stimulate the phosphorylation of pre-T

cell focal adhesion kinases. Neuroendocrinology. https://doi.org/10.1159/000054324

[33] Diep P-T, Talash K, Kasabri V (2020) Hypothesis: Oxytocin is a direct COVID-19 antiviral. Med Hypotheses 145:110329

[34] Chittepu VCSR, Kalhotra P, Osorio-Gallardo T, Jiménez-Martínez C, Robles-de la Torre RR, Gallardo-Velazquez T, Osorio-Revilla G (2019) New Molecular Insights into the Inhibition of Dipeptidyl Peptidase-4 by Natural Cyclic Peptide Oxytocin. Molecules 24:3887

[35] Akay AS, Arısan V, Cevher E, Sessevmez M, Cam B (2020) Oxytocin-loaded sustained-release hydrogel graft provides accelerated bone formation: An experimental rat study. J Orthop Res. https://doi.org/10.1002/jor.24607

[36] Oppong-Damoah A, Zaman RU, D'Souza MJ, Murnane KS (2019) Nanoparticle encapsulation increases the brain penetrance and duration of action of intranasal oxytocin. Horm Behav. https://doi.org/10.1016/j.yhbeh.2018.12.011

[37] Hua S, Vaughan B (2019) In vitro comparison of liposomal drug delivery systems targeting the oxytocin receptor: A potential novel treatment for obstetric complications. Int J Nanomedicine. https://doi.org/10.2147/IJN.S198116

Chapter 3

Oxytocin as a Metabolic Modulator

Neeru Bhatt

Abstract

Oxytocin (9-amino acid peptide) hormone is a member of the G-protein coupled receptor family. It regulates a range of physiologic actions in mammals other than assisting parturition and lactation functions. Evidence indicates that oxytocin alters lipids, protein, and sugar metabolism through various ways including modulation of appetite and satiety, enzyme activity, cellular signals, secretion of metabolic hormones, and energy consumption. Alterations in these processes have the potential to shift developmental trajectories and influence disease processes. Oxytocin can be a potential avenue for the treatment of endocrine disorders such as obesity, diabetes mellitus, and associated disorders. The chapter will include a comprehensive study about oxytocin and its physiological and pathological functions, which makes it a potential target for drug therapy.

Keywords: Oxytocin, metabolism, endocrine system, obesity, energy balance

1. Introduction

Oxytocin, which was long thought to be a hormone exclusively involved in social bonding, parturition, and lactation; now is extensively researched for its other possible implications. Evidence indicates that oxytocin alters lipid, protein, and sugar metabolism through various ways including modulation of appetite and satiety, enzyme activity, cellular signals, secretion of metabolic hormones, and energy consumption [1, 2].

1.1 Oxytocin synthesis and secretion

Oxytocin (Oxt) a nonapeptide hormone is a member of the G-protein coupled receptor family. It regulates a range of physiologic actions in mammals other than reproductive deeds [3]. The word oxytocin was taken from the Greek words (ω k ν ξ, τ o k ox ξ) meaning "quick birth". The uterine-contracting property of oxytocin was discovered by Dale [4], whereas the milk ejection property of oxytocin was revealed in the following years [5, 6].

Oxytocin is composed of nine amino acids (Cys-Tyr-Ile-Gln-Asn-Cys-Pro-Leu-GlyNH2) with a disulphide bridge between cysteine residues 1 and 6 [7, 8]. It is predominantly synthesized in magnocellular neurons of the hypothalamic paraventricular (PVN) and supraoptic (SON) nuclei of the brain. It is released into the blood circulation through the posterior pituitary gland where it is released to regulate parturition and lactation. In addition, oxytocin is produced and released outside the nervous system, such as the gastrointestinal tract [9] and bone marrow osteoblasts [10, 11] liver, placenta, amnion, heart [12], and subcutaneous adipose tissue. In adipose tissue, oxytocin has autocrine and paracrine effects via oxytocin receptors [9, 10, 13]. A variety of stimuli such as parturition, suckling, and certain stresses are responsible for the release of oxytocin in the circulation.

Endogenous oxytocin does not readily cross the blood–brain barrier, but circulating oxytocin may directly enter the hindbrain or act on the vagus nerve [14–17]. Oxytocin can enter into the cerebrospinal fluid (CSF), as proved in an animal study [18]. A significant amount of oxytocin was found in cerebrospinal fluid when copious amounts of oxytocin were injected intravenously or intranasally in nonhuman primates [18]. Additionally, exogenous oxytocin administration may accelerate endogenous oxytocin secretion either directly through PVN oxytocin autoreceptors or indirectly through peripheral oxytocin receptors [19, 20]. Generally, oxytocin receptors are found throughout the central nervous system including the hypothalamus, basal ganglia, VTA, nucleus accumbens, frontal cortex, insula, NTS, and spinal cord. Oxytocin receptors are also present in peripheral regions (vagus nerve, anterior pituitary gland, adipocytes, gastrointestinal tract, and pancreas) that regulate food intake and metabolism [12, 21–25]. Infect, mRNA for oxytocin and its receptors throughout the entire human gastrointestinal (GI) tract was recently found. Such receptors are known as allosteric modulators [12] (**Figure 1**).

1.2 The therapeutic potential of oxytocin

The therapeutic potential of oxytocin has been studied extensively for the last few years. Use of oxytocin in the treatment of autism spectrum disorder (ASD) [26, 27], schizophrenia [26, 28], and obesity [20, 28–31] have been investigated and documented in leading journals. It has opened a new door for many more untouched aspects of oxytocin to be disclosed. Recently it was found that oxytocin could reverse the effects of beta-amyloid on mice hippocampal LTP in an *in vitro* study. ERK phosphorylation and Ca^{2+}-permeable AMPA receptors are involved in this effect of oxytocin [32]. Beta-amyloid is the main culprit of Alzheimer's disease, which gets deposited around the neurons of the brain and impaired cognitive functions.

1.3 Physiological role of oxytocin in feeding regulation

Oxytocin exerts a direct as well as an indirect effect on metabolism and energy balance. The direct effect is through anorexigenic activity with increased oxytocin secretion and/or signaling leading to decreased food intake via net effects on multiple different homeostatic and neurobehavioral pathways. Peripheral oxytocin induces anorexia was first demonstrated by Arletti et al. [33]. The indirect effect of oxytocin is explicitly on muscles potentiating the majority of the slow-twitch muscles.

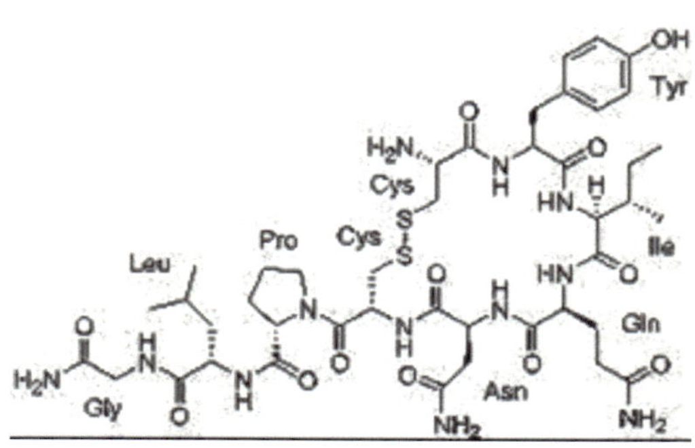

Figure 1.
Chemical structure of oxytocin [26].

Oxytocin not only affects food intake but also the choice of food that is consumed. Studies conducted with a variety of animal models, including rats, mice, and rhesus monkeys fed with standard chow with a substantial proportion of calories from carbohydrates. Such studies have shown that oxytocin reduced intake of sucrose [34–36], glucose, fructose-sweetened beverages), and HFDs sweetened with sucrose [19, 20, 30, 37–39], sucrose appears to activate a greater proportion of PVN oxytocin neurons relative to intake of fat (intralipid) [40]. Oxytocin has also been shown to suppress energy intake in animals fed HFDs without sucrose. Moreover, systemic administration of oxytocin antagonists (readily crosses the blood–brain barrier) [41] stimulates the intake of sucrose, but not chow or intralipid [42]. Conversely, impairments of oxytocin signaling is associated with increased consumption of carbohydrates, including sucrose [34, 43, 44], and glucose [44], as well as fat [38, 45], implicating a potential physiological role for oxytocin to limit consumption of both simple sugars and fat.

Oxytocin has a profound effect in termination of the food intake. The food intake is physiologically regulated by oxytocin neurons, responding to fasting and satiety conditions. It has been observed that food consumption activates oxytocin neurons [40, 46], whereas fasting is known to depress oxytocin neurons and recovery is possible with refeeding [29] or the leptin administration [47], conversely suppression of exocytosis of oxytocin, or genetic reduction of oxytocin expression increases food intake [29], and ablation of oxytocin neurons increase body weight gain by decreasing energy expenditure in male mice fed a high-fat diet (HFD) [48]. The ablation of the neurons that express oxytocin receptors, in the nucleus of the solitary tract (NTS) and arcuate nucleus induces hyperphagia [49, 50] and satiety [51]. Additionally, oxytocin also displays a circadian rhythmic pattern with a rise of circulating oxytocin level during the day and vice versa [52, 53].

1.4 The metabolic functions of oxytocin

Oxytocin is a potent regulator of caloric intake and metabolism. Metabolism is an exclusive attribute of living cells. Disturbance in metabolism can have a toll on both body and mind. Although, the epidemics of metabolic diseases have largely been attributed to genetic makeup, changes in diet, exercise and aging. However, other environmental factors may contribute to the rapid increase in the incidences.

Oxytocin has a direct effect on adipose tissue. It induces adipose tissue lipolysis [16, 20] and fat oxidation [20, 30, 54], subsequently leading to reduced body fat and weight gain [20] as well as glucose intolerance and insulin resistance. Moreover, oxytocin is believed to reduce visceral and liver fat deposition [30]. Such deposits are metabolically important and are known to increase the prognosis of metabolic syndrome and cardiovascular disease [55]. Sub chronic treatment of oxytocin extended improved adipocyte differentiation and increased gene expression of factors involved in adipogenesis in rats. This effect is related to an increased fatty acid-binding protein, peroxisome proliferator-activated receptor gamma, insulin-sensitive glucose transporter 4, leptin, and CD31 mRNA levels [56].

1.5 Energy balance

Energy balance is a complex physiological process that is regulated by multiple interactions between the gastrointestinal tract (GIT), adipose tissue, and the central nervous system (CNS). It requires both afferent signals from the periphery about the state of the energy stores as well as different signals that influence energy intake and expenditure [57] and is also influenced by behavioral, sensorial, autonomic, nutritional, and endocrine mechanisms [58]. Energy balance is quite essential in daily life to be in shape physically as well as metabolically. Nevertheless, at times energy balance (intake and expenditure) may alter partially or completely, leading to consequent pathological changes in body weight. Adaptations to body weight changes include modifications at the level of circulating appetite-related hormones that, in turn, may profoundly interact with the homeostatic and hedonistic neural centers. The homeostatic control system makes it possible to maintain energy reserves through signals of hunger stimulation that are usually downregulated when the body receives an adequate caloric intake. However, this homeostatic system is asymmetrical, showing greater effectiveness in defending against energy deficit in the light of reduced efficiency in the defense against the energy excess. Furthermore, the homeostatic system is strongly influenced by hedonic signals, based on reward mechanisms, frequently causing food intake even in the absence of biological needs. This review will summarize the role of the main central and peripheral hormones involved in controlling energy balance.

2. Mechanisms underlying the effects of oxytocin on energy balance

The proposed mechanisms underlying the effects of oxytocin on calorie balance are discussed under the following topics.

2.1 Oxytocin may regulate appetite

Oxytocin may induce satiety by slowing gastric emptying [59–61]. Gastric emptying is a principal trait of postprandial glycemia. A lower rate of gastric emptying and a high-fat diet rationally enhances the glycemic index of carbohydrates. Moreover, slowing of gastric emptying by fat depends on the small intestine exposed to lipolytic products. Oxytocin is released in response to a fatty meal [62], which regulates gastric emptying [63, 64].

Conversely, systemic administration of oxytocin led to enhanced gastric emptying [63, 64] also oxytocin receptor antagonist atosiban delayed gastric emptying significantly [9]. Though the results from human studies are conflicting and only one human study on diabetic gastroparesis has reported prolonged gastric emptying time (40–80 mIU/min) [65]. The prokinetic effect of oxytocin on the gut has been assumed to be similar to the one in uterine myometrium and mammary myoepithelial cells; i.e., the intracellular release of **Ca2+** which leads to muscle contraction via myosin light kinase activity [12]. In normal subjects, oxytocin has been found in the gut where it is secreted after a meal [62] and stimulates colonic activity [66].

Oxytocin can influence other appetite-regulating hormones. Intravenous administration of oxytocin modulated levels of ghrelin (which is orexigenic) in human subjects [67], whereas 24 IU intranasal administration of oxytocin did not show any significant changes in fasting or postprandial levels of ghrelin [68, 69]. Ghrelin is a gastric hormone, which regulates hunger and food intake. Likewise, oxytocin administration can influence cholecystokinin concentration in circulation [60] but this change was not related to differences in caloric consumption between oxytocin and placebo conditions [35]. Oxytocin facilitates cholecystokinin elicited excitation of neurons within the nucleus of the solitary tract and reduces food intake [49].

2.2 Oxytocin and glucose homeostasis

Oxytocin influences glucose and insulin homeostasis, along with bodyweight balance. Numerous studies have shown that oxytocin encourages glucose uptake [70, 71] and stimulates insulin secretion [72–76] as well as pancreatic glucagon secretion [75], which extends a hint about the involvement of oxytocin in the prognosis of diabetes. Intracerebroventricular oxytocin can improve insulin levels by activation of vagal cholinergic neurons innervating pancreatic beta-cells [76]. Conversely, insulin can modulate oxytocin levels in the hypothalamus by activating the insulin-regulated aminopeptidase as well [77, 78].

Studies have suggested that oxytocin has the capacity to reduce obesity-related diabetic changes, such as glucose intolerance, insulin resistance, and pancreatic islet hypertrophy [19, 20, 30, 38, 79, 80]. Two weeks of treatment with oxytocin decreased adiposity and food intake in obese mice lacking leptin, although, it worsens glucose metabolism, most likely due to an increase in corticosterone levels and enhanced hepatic glucose production. It could be suggested that the effect of oxytocin in decreasing fat mass is independent of leptin, while the beneficial impact on glucose metabolism requires the presence of leptin [81]. Whereas, oxytocin treatment for a longer period, notably reduced body fat accumulation, fasting blood glucose levels, and improved insulin sensitivity and glucose tolerance in leptin receptor-deficient mice [82]. The hypoglycemic stimulatory effect on insulin secretion and sensitivity, and improvement of pancreatic islet cells after oxytocin administration strongly suggested that oxytocin might be a therapeutic target for treating diabetes.

Oxytocin influences glucose metabolism in various ways. It may have a direct effect on glucose metabolism through the promotion of muscle cell differentiation. It has been found that a higher oxytocin concentration is linked with the anabolic effects of steroids in bovine and ovine skeletal muscle [83, 84]. A rapid increase in muscle regeneration was observed in old mice with a cardiotoxin muscle injury, when oxytocin was administered subcutaneously [79], though, the regenerative capacity of skeletal muscle and the levels of oxytocin receptor in muscle stem cells decrease with the age [79].

Further oxytocin-induced augmentation of muscle mass directly affects glucose uptake and insulin sensitivity. Oxytocin receptors are widely distributed in adipocytes of both humans and animals, especially in rats [12, 85, 86]. Oxytocin augments the transient increase in intracellular Ca^{2+} and stimulates PKC activity [87, 88], which in turn increases glucose uptake in mice adipocytes [88–90]. It has been noted that oxytocin stimulates glucose oxidation via enhancement of pyruvate dehydrogenase activity in mice adipocytes [90]. Oxytocin treatment induced a higher mRNA expression for gluconeogenesis and lowered glycaemia in lean control mice, probably because of the decreased liver glycogen content [82]. So, oxytocin treatment enhances net hepatic glucose oxidation, reduced glycogen synthase activity, and increased glycogen phosphorylase activity [91].

Oxytocin modulates pancreatic function centrally via vagal cholinergic neurons innervating β-cells [76] and peripherally by stimulating phosphoinositide turnover and activating PKC in pancreatic β-cells [92]. Insulin secretion (independent of glucose concentration) was found to be stimulated in isolated mouse pancreatic islets with oxytocin infusion [91]. Additionally, oxytocin increases insulin and glucagon secretion in both *in vivo* and in situ conditions and appears to have a greater effect on glucagon secretion than on insulin secretion (and to a much greater extent in insulin-deficient diabetic rats) [93–95]. Peripherally oxytocin regulates whole-body glucose metabolism. Studies have shown that oxytocin-deficient (*Oxt*$^{-/-}$) and high-fat diet-fed OTR-deficient (*Oxtr*$^{-/-}$) mice had decreased insulin sensitivity and impaired glucose tolerance [96, 97], and both insulin sensitivity, as well as glucose tolerance, were restored after oxytocin administration in obese diabetic (*db/db*) mice fed with standard and high-fat diets [20, 30, 82, 98]. Improvements in glucose tolerance, lowering of postprandial plasma glucose and insulin concentrations have been reported in subjects with normal weight and obesity who were given oxytocin [33, 68, 69, 80, 99]. In contrast, increases in plasma glucose and hepatic glycogenolytic activity concurrent with an absence of effects on peripheral insulin sensitivity have also been reported [95].

2.3 The lipolytic effect of oxytocin

The lipolytic effect of oxytocin is well studied in animal models [16, 20] and human trials [100]. The intravenous administration of oxytocin (10 mIU/kg) increased plasma levels of non-esterified free fatty acids and reduced plasma levels of triglycerides in women with obese history [100]. Even the intranasal administration of oxytocin (24 IU before meals and at bedtime) in overweight or obese men and women for eight weeks resulted in improved lipid profile (lower levels of total cholesterol and LDL cholesterol), reduced waist circumference, and weight loss [80]. Oxytocin also acts as a homeostatic inhibitor of consumption, capable of mitigating multiple aspects of consumption behavior and energy metabolism [34]. Markedly, oxytocin reduces metabolically important fat for instance visceral and liver fat [30]. Such fat deposits are mostly responsible for the increased risk of metabolic syndrome and cardiovascular disease [55].

2.4 Energy expenditure

Despite the weight loss, it is believed that oxytocin contributed to the preservation of lean body mass, a key determinant of energy expenditure [54], activation of brown fat [97, 101, 102] and conversion of white adipose tissue to beige fat that is capable of thermogenesis [68, 82]. In young female athletes and non-athletes aged 14–21 years, fasting levels of oxytocin were positively associated with resting energy expenditure [68].

3. Conclusions

Metabolic disorders have reached to an explosive level and data projected by different government or non-government bodies are scary. Some alternative treatments should be adopted other than the conventional mode of treatment to coping such situations. Hormones are very powerful chemical substances and work precisely in the target organ. They mostly secrete far away from the site of action. Oxytocin is one such hormone that was long known for its reproductive involvement and is now being investigated for its multifunctional attributes. The therapeutic implications of oxytocin are gaining momentum. Studies have revealed that oxytocin alters metabolism in various ways including modulation of appetite and satiety, enzyme activity, cellular signals, secretion of hormones, and energy consumption. Despite the wealth of basic research showing broad anorexigenic effects of oxytocin, clinical studies on oxytocin's therapeutic potential in obesity, and associated disorders are still in their infancy and exhaustive research is needed. Future replicated and validated studies will help to characterize and better understand the underlying mechanisms for the regulation/dysregulation of metabolism and would be a good approach for treating the obese population, which is the need of the hour.

Acknowledgements

All the researchers and authors referred and cited here are duly acknowledged.

Conflict of interest

The author declares no conflict of interest, financial or otherwise.

Other declarations

I am grateful to IOOS Programme of Intech Open for waiving publication fees completely.

Acronyms and abbreviations

AMP	Adenosine monophosphate
Ca	calcium
CD31	The cell adhesion molecule
CSF	Cerebrospinal fluid
CVD	Cardio vascular diseases
ERK	Extracellular signal-regulated kinase
HFDs	High fructose syrup
LDL	Low density lipoprotein
LTPL	Long term potentiation(hippocampus)
mRNA	Messenger RNA
NTS	Nucleus tractus solitarius
PKC	Protein kinase
PVN	paraventricular
VTA	Ventral tegmental area

Author details

Neeru Bhatt
Canadian Journal of Clinical Nutrition, Global Science Heritage, Ontario, Canada

*Address all correspondence to: neerubhattdp@gmail.com

References

[1] Ding C, Leow MKS, Magkos F. Oxytocin in metabolic homeostasis: implications for obesity and diabetes management. Obes Rev. 2019;20(1):22-40. doi: 10.1111/obr.12757.

[2] Sabatier N, Leng G, Menzies J. Oxytocin, feeding, and satiety, Fronti Endocrl. 2013; 4: 35.

[3] Meyer-Lindenberg A, Domes G, Kirsch P, Heinrichs M. Oxytocin and vasopressin in the human brain: social neuropeptides for translational medicine. Nat Rev Neurosci. 2011; 12: 524-538.

[4] Dale HH. On some physiological actions of ergot. J Physio. 1906; 34:163-206.

[5] Ott I, Scott JC. The Action of Infundibulum upon Mammary Secretion. Proc Soc Exp Biol. 1910; 8: 48-49.

[6] Schafer EA, Mackenzie K. The action of animal extracts on milk secretion. Proceedings of the Royal Society of London Series B-Containing Papers of a Biological Character. 1911; 84:16-22.

[7] du Vigneaud V, Ressler C, Trippett S. The sequence of amino acids in oxytocin, with a proposal for the structure of oxytocin. J Biol Chem. 1953b; 205:949-957.

[8] Tuppy H. The amino-acid sequence in oxytocin. Biochim Biophys Acta. 1953; 11: 449-450.

[9] Ohlsson B, Björgell O, Ekberg O, Darwiche G. The oxytocin/vasopressin receptor antagonist atosiban delays the gastric emptying of a semisolid meal compared to saline in human. Bio Med cent Gastroenterol. 2006; 6:11. doi:10.1186/1471-230X-6-11

[10] Qin J, Feng M, Wang C, Ye Y, Wang PS, Liu C. Oxytocin receptor expressed on the smooth muscle mediates the excitatory effect of oxytocin on gastric motility in rats. Neurogastroenterl Motil. 2009; 21:430-438. doi: 10.1111/j. 1365-2982.2009. 01282.x

[11] Elabd C, Basillais A, Beaupied, H, Breuil V, Wagner N, Scheideler M, Zaragosi LE, Massiéra F, Lemichez E, Trajanoski Z, Carle G, Euller-Ziegler L, Ailhaud G, Benhamou CL, Dani C, Amri EZ. Oxytocin controls differentiation of human mesenchymal stem cells and reverses osteoporosis. Stem Cell. 2008; 26: 2399-2407.

[12] Gimpl G, Fahrenholz F. The oxytocin receptor system: structure, function, and regulation. Physiol Rev. 2001; 81:629-683.

[13] Feng M, Qin J, Wang C, Ye Y, Wang S, Xie D, Wang P S, Liu C. Estradiol upregulates the expression of oxytocin receptor in colon in rats. Am J Physiol Endocrinl Metabol. 2009; 296: E1059–E1066. doi: 10.1152/ ajpendo.90609.2008

[14] Welch MG, Tamir H, Gershon MD. Expression and developmental regulation of oxytocin (OT) and oxytocin receptors (OTR) in the enteric nervous system (ENS) and intestinal epithelium. J Compar Neur. 2009; 512:256-270. doi: 10.1002/cne.21872

[15] Ho JM, Anekonda VT, Thompson BW, Zhu M, Curry RW, Hwang B H, Morton GJ, Schwartz MW, Baskin DG, Appleyard SM, Blevins JE. Hindbrain oxytocin receptors contribute to the effects of circulating oxytocin on food intake in male rats. Endocrinl. 2014; 155:2845-2857. doi: 10.1210/ en.2014-1148

[16] Blevins JE, Graham JL, Morton GJ, Bales KL, Schwartz MW, Baskin DG, Havel PJ. Chronic oxytocin

administration inhibits food intake, increases energy expenditure, and produces weight loss in fructose-fed obese rhesus monkeys. Am J Physiol Regul Integ Comparat Physiol. 2015; 308(5): R431-R438. doi: 10.1152/ajpregu.00441.2014.

[17] Iwasaki Y, Maejima Y, Suyama S, Yoshida M, Arai T, Katsurada K, Kumari P, Nakabayashi H, Kakei M, Yada T. Peripheral oxytocin activates vagal afferent neurons to suppress feeding in normal and leptin-resistant mice: a route for ameliorating hyperphagia and obesity. Am J Physiol Regul Integ Comparat Physiol. 2015;308: R360–R369. doi: 10.1152/ajpregu.00344.2014

[18] Lee MR, Scheidweiler KB, Diao XX, Akhlaghi F, Cummins A, Huestis MA, Leggio L, Averbeck BB. Oxytocin by intranasal and intravenous routes reaches the cerebrospinal fluid in rhesus macaques: determination using a novel oxytocin assay. Mol Psychiat. 2017; 23(1):115-122.

[19] Zhang G, Cai D. Circadian intervention of obesity development via resting stage feeding manipulation or oxytocin treatment. Am J Physiol Endocrinl Metab. 2011; 301: E1004–E1012. doi:10.1152/ajpendo.00196.2011

[20] Deblon N, Veyrat-Durebex C, Bourgoin L, Caillon A, Bussier AL, Petrosino S, Piscitelli F, Legros JJ, Geenen V, Foti M. Wahli W, Di Marzo V, Rohner-Jeanrenaud F. Mechanisms of the anti-obesity effects of oxytocin in diet-induced obese rats. Pub Lib Sci One. 2011; 6(9): e25565. doi: 10.1371/journal.pone.0025565

[21] Blevins JE, Baskin DG. Translational and therapeutic potential of oxytocin as an anti-obesity strategy: Insights from rodents, nonhuman primates and humans. Physiol Behav. 2015; 152 (Pt B):438-449. doi: 10.1016/j.physbeh.2015.05.023.

[22] Qian W, Zhu T, Tang B Yu S, Hu H, Sun W, Pan R, Wang J, Wang D, Yang L, Mao C, Zhou L, Yuan G. Decreased circulating levels of oxytocin in obesity and newly diagnosed type 2 diabetic patients. J Clin Endocrinl Metab. 2014; 99: 4683– 4689.

[23] Feng Y, Kapormai K, Barr CL. Association of the GABRD gene and childhood - onset mood disorders. Genes Brain Behav. 2010; 9(6):668-672.

[24] Gould BR, Zingg HH. Mapping oxytocin receptor gene expression in the mouse brain and mammary gland using an oxytocin receptor-LacZ reporter mouse. Neurosci. 2003; 122:155-167

[25] Antoni FA. Oxytocin receptors in rat adenohypophysis: evidence from radioligand binding studies. Endocrinl. 1986; 119:2393-2395. doi: 10.1210/endo-119-5-2393

[26] Striepens N, Kendrick KM, Maier W, Hurlemann R. Prosocial effects of oxytocin and clinical evidence for its therapeutic potential. [Research Support, Non-U.S. Gov't Review]. Front Neuroendocrinl. 2011; 32(4): 426-450. doi: 10.1016/j.yfrne.2011.07.001.

[27] Yamasue H, Yee JR, Hurlemann R, Rilling JK, Chen FS, Meyer Lindenberg A, et al. Integrative approaches utilizing oxytocin to enhance prosocial behavior: from animal and human social behavior to autistic social dysfunction. J Neurosci. 2012; 32(41):14109-14117. doi:10.1523/JNEUROSCI.3327-12.2012.

[28] Montag C, Brockmann EM, Bayerl M, Rujescu D, Muller DJ, Gallinat J. Oxytocin and oxytocin receptor gene polymorphisms and risk for schizophrenia: A case–control study. World J Biol Psychi. 2012; 14(7): 500-508. doi:10.3109/15622975.2012.677547.

[29] Kublaoui BM, Gemelli T, Tolson KP, Wang Y, Zinn AR. Oxytocin deficiency mediates hyperphagic obesity of Sim1 haplo insufficient mice. Mol Endocrinl 2008; 22: 1723-1734.

[30] Maejima Y, Iwasaki Y, Yamahara Y, Kodaira M, Sedbazar U, Yada T. Peripheral oxytocin treatment ameliorates obesity by reducing food intake and visceral fat mass. Aging (Albany NY). 2011; 3(12):1169-1177.

[31] Maejima Y, Sedbazar U, Suyama S, Kohno D, Onaka T, Takano E, Yoshida N, Koike M, Uchiyama Y, Fujiwara K, Yashiro T, Horvath TL, Dietrich MO, Tanaka S, Dezaki K, Oh S, Hashimoto K, Shimizu H, Nakata M, Mori M, Yada T. Nesfatin-1-regulated oxytocinergic signaling in the paraventricular nucleus causes anorexia through a leptin independent melanocortin pathway. [Research Support, N.I.H., Extramural Research Support, Non-U.S. Gov't]. Cell Metab. 2009; 10(5): 355-365. doi: 10.1016/j. cmet.2009.09.002.

[32] Takahashi J, Yamada D, Ueta Y, Iwai T, Koga E, Tanabe M, Oka JI, Saitoh A. Oxytocin reverses Aβ-induced impairment of hippocampal synaptic plasticity in mice. Bioche Biophy Res Commun. 2020; 528 (1): 174-178. doi: 10.1016/j.bbrc.2020.04.046

[33] Arletti R, Benelli A, Bertolini A. Influence of oxytocin on feeding behavior in the rat. Peptides. 1989; 10: 89– 93

[34] Olszewski PK, Klockars A, Schioth HB, Levine AS. Oxytocin as feeding inhibitor: maintaining homeostasis in consummatory behavior. Pharmacol Biochem Behav. 2010; 97: 47-54.

[35] Amico JA, Vollmer RR, Cai HM, Miedlar JA, Rinaman L. Enhanced initial and sustained intake of sucrose solution in mice with an oxytocin gene deletion. [Research Support, N.I.H., Extramural]. Am J Physiol Regul Integr Comp Physiol. 2005; 289(6): R1798–R1806. doi:10.1152/ajpregu. 00558.2005.

[36] Sclafani A, Rinaman L, Vollmer RR, Amico JA. Oxytocin knockout mice demonstrate enhanced intake of sweet and nonsweet carbohydrate solutions. Am J Physiol Regul Integr Comp Physiol. 2007; 292(5): R1828–R1833. doi:10.1152/ajpregu.00826.2006

[37] Mullis K, Kay K, Williams DL. Oxytocin action in the ventral tegmental area affects sucrose intake. Brain Res. 2013; 1513: 1585-1591.

[38] Zhang G, Bai H, Zhang H, Dean C, Wu Q, Li J, Guariglia S, Meng Q, Cai D. Neuropeptide exocytosis involving synaptotagmin-4 and oxytocin in hypothalamic programming of body weight and energy balance. Neuron. 2011; 69:523-535. doi:10.1016/j. neuron.2010.12.036 29.

[39] Morton GJ, Thatcher BS, Reidelberger RD, Ogimoto K, Wolden Hanson T, Baskin DG, Schwartz MW, Blevins JE. Peripheral oxytocin suppresses food intake and causes weight loss in diet-induced obese rats. Am J Physiol Endocrinl Metab. 2012; 302: E134 –E144.

[40] Johnstone LE, Fong TM, Leng G. Neuronal activation in the hypothal amus and brainstem during feeding in rats. Cell Metab. 2006; 4: 313-321.

[41] Boccia ML, Goursaud AP, Bachevalier J, Anderson KD, Pedersen CA. Peripherally administered non-peptide oxytocin antagonist, L368,899, accumulates in limbic brain areas: a new pharmacological tool for the study of social motivation in non-human primates. Horm Behav. 2007; 52(3): 344-351. doi: 10.1016/j. yhbeh.2007. 05.009.

[42] Olszewski PK, Klockars A, Olszewska AM, Fredriksson R, Schioth HB, Levine AS. Molecular, immunohistochemical, and pharmacological evidence of oxytocin's role as inhibitor of carbohydrate but not fat intake. Endocrinl. 2010; 151(10): 4736-4744. doi: 10.1210/en.2010-0151.

[43] Amico JA, Vollmer RR, Cai HM, Miedlar JA, Rinaman L. Enhanced initial and sustained intake of sucrose solution in mice with an oxytocin gene deletion. Am J Physiol Regul Integr Comp Physiol. 2005; 289: R1798 –R1806.

[44] Herisson FM, Brooks LL, Waas JR, Levine AS, Olszewski PK. Functional relationship between oxytocin and appetite for carbohydrates versus saccharin. Neuroreport. 2014; 25: 909 –914.

[45] Zhang G, Bai H, Cai D. Neuropeptide exocytosis involving synaptotagmin-4 and oxytocin in hypothalamic programming of body weight and energy balance. Neuron. 2011; 69: 523– 535.

[46] Hume C, Sabatier N, Menzies J. High-sugar, but not high-fat, food activates supraoptic nucleus neurons in the male rat. Endocrinl. 2017; 158: 2200-2211.

[47] Tung YCL, Ma M, Piper S, Coll A, O'Rahilly S, Yeo GS. Novel leptin-regulated genes revealed by transcriptional profiling of the hypothalamic paraventricular nucleus. J Neurosci. 2008; 28:12419-12426.

[48] Wu Z, Xu Y, Zhu Y, Sutton AK, Zhao R, Lowell BB, Olson DP, Tong Q. An obligate role of oxytocin neurons in diet induced energy expenditure. Pub Lib Sci One. 2012; 7: e45167. doi: 10.1371 /journal. pone. 0045167

[49] Baskin DG, Kim F, Gelling RW, Russell BJ, Schwartz MW, Morton GJ, Simhan HN, Moralejo DH, Blevins JE. A new oxytocin-saporin cytotoxin for lesioning oxytocin-receptive neurons in the rat hindbrain. Endocrinl. 2010; 151: 4207-4213

[50] Ong ZY, Bongiorno DM, Hernando MA, Grill HJ. Effects of endogenous oxytocin receptor signaling in nucleus tractus solitarius on satiation-mediated feeding and thermogenic control in male rats. Endocrinl. 2017; 158: 2826-2836.

[51] Fenselau H, Campbell JN, Verstegen AM, Madara JC, Xu J, Shah BP, Resch JM, Yang Z, Mandelblat-Cerf Y, Livneh Y, Lowell BB. A rapidly acting glutamatergic ARC→PVH satiety circuit postsynaptically regulated by αMSH. Nat Neurosci. 2017; 20: 42-51

[52] Zhang G, Bai H, Zhang H, Dean C, Wu Q, Li J, Guairglia S, Meng Q, Cai D. Neuropeptide exocytosis involving synaptotagmin-4 and oxytocin in hypothalamic programming of body weight and energy balance. Neuron. 2011; 69: 523– 535.

[53] Maejima Y, Takahashi S, Takasu K, Takenoshita S, Ueta Y, Shimomura K. Orexin action on oxytocin neurons in the paraventricular nucleus of the hypothalamus. Neuroreport. 2017; 28: 360-366

[54] Blevins JE, Thompson BW, Anekonda VT, Ho JM, Graham JL, Roberts ZS, Hwang BH, Ogimoto K, Wolden-Hanson T, Nelson J, Kaiyala KJ, Havel PJ, Bales KL, Morton GJ, Schwartz MW, Baskin DG. Chronic CNS oxytocin signaling preferentially induces fat loss in high-fat diet-fed rats by enhancing satiety responses and increasing lipid utilization. Am J Physiol Regul Integrat Comparat Physiol. 2016; 310: R640–R658. doi: 10.1152/ ajpregu.00220.2015.

[55] Pischon T, Boeing H, Hoffmann K, Bergmann M, Schulze MB, Overvad K,

van der Schouw YT, Spencer E, Moons KGM, Tjønneland A, Halkjaer J, Jensen MK, Stegger J, Clavel-Chapelon F, Boutron-Ruault MC, Chajes V, Linseisen J, Kaaks R, Trichopoulou A, Trichopoulos D, Bamia C, Sieri S, Palli D, Tumino R, Vineis P, Panico S, Peeters PHM, May AM, Bueno-de-Mesquita HB, van Duijnhoven FJB, Hallmans G, Weinehall L, Manjer J, Hedblad B, Lund E, Agudo A, Arriola L, Barricarte A, Navarro C, Martinez C, Quirós JR, Key T, Bingham S, Khaw KT, Boffetta P, Jenab M, Ferrari P, Riboli E. General and abdominal adiposity and risk of death in Europe. New Eng J Med. 2008; 359:2105-2120. doi: 10.1056/NEJMoa0801891.

[56] Hoyda D, Fry M, Ahima RS, Ferguson AV. Adiponectin selectively inhibits oxytocin neurons of the paraventricular nucleus of the hypothalamus. J Physiol. 2007; 585 (3): 805-816.

[57] Sandoval D, Cota D, Seeley RJ. The integrative role of CNS fuel-sensing mechanisms in energy balance and glucose regulation. Annu Rev Physiol. 2008; 70: 513-535

[58] Boguszewski CL, Paz-Filho G, Velloso LA. Neuroendocrine body weight regulation: integration between fat tissue, gastrointestinal tract, and the brain. Endokrynol Pol. 2010; 61, 194-206

[59] Wu CL, Hung CR, Chang FY, Pau KYF, Wang JL, Wang PS. Involvement of cholecystokinin receptor in the inhibition of gastric emptying by oxytocin in male rats. Pflugers Arch. 2002; 445:187-193. doi: 10.1007/s00424-002-0925-7.

[60] Wu CL, Hung CR, Chang FY, Pau KYF, Wang PS. Pharmacological effects of oxytocin on gastric emptying and intestinal transit of a non-nutritive liquid meal in female rats, Naunyn-Schmiedeberg's Arc Pharmacol. 2003; 367 (4): 406-413

[61] Rogers RC, Hermann GE. Oxytocin, oxytocin antagonist, TRH, and hypothalamic paraventricular nucleus stimulation effects on gastric motility. Peptides. 1987; 8:505-513. http://doi.org/10.1016/0196-9781(87)90017-9.

[62] Ohlsson B, Forsling ML, Rehfeld JF, Sjölund K: Cholecystokinin leads to increased oxytocin secretion in healthy women. Eur J Surg. 2002; 168:114-118.

[63] Hashmonai M, Torem S, Argov S, Barzilai A, Schramek A: Prolonged post-vagotomy gastric atony treated by oxytocin. Br J Surg. 1979; 66:550-551.

[64] Petring OU. The effect of oxytocin on basal and pethidine-induced delayed gastric emptying. Br J Clin Pharmacol. 1989; 28:329-332.

[65] Borg J, Ohlsson B. Oxytocin prolongs the gastric emptying time in patients with diabetes mellitus and gastroparesis, but does not affect satiety or volume intake in patients with functional dyspepsia. Bio Med Centr Res Notes. 2012; 5:148. doi: 10.1186/1756-0500-5-148.

[66] Ohlsson B, Ringström G, Abrahamsson H, Simrén M, Björnsson ES. Oxytocin stimulates colonic motor activity in healthy women. Neurogastroenterol Mot. 2004; 16:233-240

[67] Schorr M, Marengi DA, Pulumo RL, Yu E, Eddy KT, Klibanski A, Miller KK, Lawson EA. Oxytocin and its relationship to bone mineral density and hip geometry across the weight spectrum. J Clin Endocrinol Metabol. 2017; 102:2814-2824.

[68] Lawson EA, Marengi DA, DeSanti RL, Holmes TM, Schoenfeld DA, Tolley CJ. Oxytocin

reduces caloric intake in men. Obesity. 2015; 23: 950-956.

[69] Ott V, Finlayson G, Lehnert H et al. Oxytocin reduces reward-driven food intake in humans. Diabetes. 2013; 62: 3418-3425.

[70] Florian M, Jankowski M, Gutkowska J. Oxytocin increases glucose uptake in neonatal rat cardiomyocytes. Endocrinl. 2010; 151(2):482-491. doi:10.1210/ en.2009-0624

[71] Lee ES, Uhm KO, Lee YM, Kwon J, Park SH, Soo KH. Oxytocin stimulates glucose uptake in skeletal muscle cells through the calcium-CaMKK-AMPK pathway. Regul Pept. 2008; 151(1-3):71-74. doi: 10.1016/j.regpep.2008.05.001

[72] Knudtzon J. Acute effects of oxytocin and vasopressin on plasma levels of glucagon, insulin and glucose in rabbits. Horm Metab Res. 1983; 15:103-104. doi:10.1055/s-2007-

[73] Chiodera P, Coiro V, Camellini L, Rossi G, Pignatti D, Volpi R, Roti E. Effect of pharmacological doses of oxytocin on insulin response to glucose in normal man. Horm Res. 1984; 20(2):150-154. doi:10.1159/000179988

[74] Paolisso G, Sgambato S, Giugliano D, Pizza G, Tesauro P, Varricchio M, D'Onofrio F. Effects of oxytocin delivery on counter-regulatory hormone response in insulin dependent (type 1) diabetic subjects. Horm Res. 1989; 31:250-255. doi:10.1159/000181126

[75] Altszuler N, Winkler B, Rosenberg CR, Pi-Sunyer FX, Fuchs AR. Role of insulin and glucagon in oxytocin effects on glucose metabolism. Proc Soc Exp Biol Med. 1992; 199(2):236-242. doi:10.3181/00379727-199-43353

[76] Björkstrand E, Eriksson M, Uvnäs-Moberg K. Evidence of a peripheral and a central effect of oxytocin on pancreatic hormone release in rats. Neuroendocrinl. 1996; 63(4): 377-383. doi:10.1159/000126978

[77] Fernando RN, Larm J, Albiston AL, Chai SY. Distribution and cellular localization of insulin-regulated aminopeptidase in the rat central nervous system. J Comparative Neurol. 2005; 487 (4): 372-390

[78] Zambotti-Villela L, Yamasaki SC, Villarroel JS, Alponti RF, Silveira PF. Aspartyl, arginyl and alanyl aminopeptidase activities in the hippocampus and hypothalamus of streptozotocin-induced diabetic rats. Brain Res. 2007; 1170:112-118.

[79] Elabd C, Cousin W, Upadhyay P, Chen RY, Chooljian MS, Li J, Kung S, Jiang KP, Conboy IM. Oxytocin is an age-specific circulating hormone that is necessary for muscle maintenance and regeneration. Nat Commun. 2014; 5: 4082.

[80] Zhang H, Wu C, Chen Q, Chen X, Xu Z, Wu J, et al. Treatment of obesity and diabetes using oxytocin or analogs in patients and mouse models. Pub Lib Sci One. 2013; 8(5): e61477. doi: 10.1371/journal.pone.0061477

[81] Altirriba J, Poher AL, Caillon A, Arsenijevic D, Veyrat-Durebex C, Lyautey J, Dulloo A, Rohner-Jeanrenaud F. Divergent effects of oxytocin treatment of obese diabetic mice on adiposity and diabetes. Endocrinl. 2014; 155(11):4189-4201. doi:10.1210/ en.2014-1466

[82] Plante E, Menaouar A, Danalache BA, Yip D, Broderick TL, Chiasson JL, Jankowski M, Gutkowska J. Oxytocin treatment prevents the cardiomyopathy observed in obese diabetic male db/db mice. Endocrinl. 2015; 156(4):1416-1428. doi:10.1210/ en.2014- 1718

[83] Jager ND, Hudson NJ, Reverter A, Wang YH, Nagaraj SH, Café L M,

Greenwood PL, Barnard RT, Kongsuwan KP, Dalrymple BP. Chronic exposure to anabolic steroids induces the muscle expression of oxytocin and a more than fiftyfold increase in circulating oxytocin in cattle. Physiol Genom. 2011; 43: 467-478.

[84] Kongsuwan K, Knox MR, Allingham PG, Pearson R, Dalrymple BP. The effect of combination treatment with trenbolone acetate and estradiol-17β on skeletal muscle expression and plasma concentrations of oxytocin in sheep. Domest Anim Endocrinl. 2012; 43: 67-73.

[85] Tsuda T, Ueno Y, Yoshikawa T, Kojo H, Osawa T. Microarray profiling of gene expression in human adipocytes in response to anthocyanins. Biochem Pharmacol. 2006; 71: 1184-1197.

[86] Gajdosechova L, Krskova K, Segarra AB, Spolcova A, Suski M, Olszanecki R, Zorad S. Hypooxyto cinaemia in obese Zucker rats relates to oxytocin degradation in liver and adipose tissue. J Endocrinl. 2014; 220: 333-343.

[87] Schwartz Y, Goodman HM, Yamaguchi H. Refractoriness to growth hormone is associated with increased intracellular calcium in rat adipocytes. Proc Natl Acad Sci U S A. 1991; 88: 6790– 6794

[88] Egan JJ, Saltis J, Wek SA, Simpson IA, Londos C. Insulin, oxytocin, and vasopressin stimulate protein kinase C activity in adipocyte plasma membranes. Proc Natl Acad Sci U S A. 1990; 87: 1052– 1056.

[89] Mühlbacher C, Karnieli E, Schaff P, Obermaier B, Mushack J, Rattenhuber E, Häring HU. Phorbol esters imitate in rat fat-cells the full effect of insulin on glucose-carrier translocation, but not on 3-O-methylglucose-transport activity. Biochem J. 1988; 249: 865– 870.

[90] Mukherjee SP, Mukherjee C. Stimulation of pyruvate dehydrogenase activity in adipocytes by oxytocin: evidence for mediation of the insulin-like effect by endogenous hydrogen peroxide independent of glucose transport. Arch Biochem Biophys. 1982; 214: 211– 222.

[91] Arino J, Bosch F, Gomez-Foix AM, Guinovart JJ. Oxytocin inactivates and phosphorylates rat hepatocyte glycogen synthase. Biochem J. 1989; 261: 827– 830.

[92] Gao ZY, Drews G, Henquin JC. Mechanisms of the stimulation of insulin release by oxytocin in normal mouse islets. Biochem J. 1991; 276: 169-174.

[93] Dunning BE, Moltz JH, Fawcett CP. Modulation of insulin and glucagon secretion from the perfused rat pancreas by the neurohypophysial hormones and by desamino-D-arginine vasopressin (DDAVP). Peptides. 1984; 5: 871– 875.

[94] Widmaier EP, Shah PR, Lee G. Interactions between oxytocin, glucagon and glucose in normal and streptozotocin-induced diabetic rats. Regul Pept. 1991; 34: 235– 249.

[95] Paolisso G, Pizza G, De Riu S, Marrazzo G, Sgambato S, Giugliano D, Varricchio M, D'Onofrio F. Effects of oxytocin upon the endocrine pancreas secretion and glucose turnover in normal man. Eur J Endocrinl. 1990; 123: 504– 510.

[96] Camerino C. Low sympathetic tone and obese phenotype in oxytocin deficient mice. Obesity. 2009; 17: 980 –984.

[97] Watanabe S, Wei FY, Matsunaga T, Matsunaga N, Kaitsuka T, Tomizawa K. Oxytocin protects against

stress-induced cell death in murine pancreatic β-cells. Sci Rep. 2016; 6: 25185.

[98] Mohan S, Khan D, Moffett RC, Irwin N, Flatt PR. Oxytocin is present in islets and plays a role in beta-cell function and survival. Peptides. 2018; 100: 260– 268.

[99] Klement J, Ott V, Rapp K, Brede S, Piccinini F, Cobelli C, Lehnert H, Hallschmid M. Oxytocin improves beta-cell responsivity and glucose tolerance in healthy men. Diabetes. 2016; 66(2): 264-271. https://doi.org/10.2337/db16-0569

[100] Burt RL, Leake NH, Dannenburg WN. Effect of synthetic oxytocin on plasma non esterified fatty acids, triglycerides, and blood glucose. Obstet Gyneco.1963; 21:708-712.

[101] Kasahara Y, Takayanagi Y, Kawada T, Itoi K, Nishimori K. Impaired thermoregulatory ability of oxytocin-deficient mice during cold-exposure. Biosci Biotechnol Biochem. 2007; 71: 3122-3126.

[102] Takayanagi Y, Kasahara Y, Onaka T, Takahashi N, Kawada T, Nishimori K. Oxytocin receptor-deficient mice developed late-onset obesity. Neuroreport. 2008; 19: 951-955.

Chapter 4

Oxytocin and Neuroprotective Effects

Oytun Erbaş and İlknur Altuntaş

Abstract

The neurohormone oxytocin (OT), consisting of nine amino acids, is produced in the hypothalamus and secreted from the posterior lobe of the pituitary gland. Recent studies show that OT can affect the course of the disease and is promising in the treatment of neurodegenerative disorders, due to its therapeutic properties and benefits. Histological and biochemical findings of the studies on vincristine-induced neuropathy, cisplatin-induced cytotoxicity, diabetic neuropathy, rotenone-induced Parkinson's disease, hypoxia, and stroke, which are reviewed in this chapter, revealed that OT significantly prevented neuronal damage with its anti-inflammatory and antioxidant properties. Therefore, the neuroprotective effects of OT and the underlying molecular mechanisms continue to attract the attention of scientists.

Keywords: oxytocin, neurohormone, neuroprotection

1. Introduction

The neurohypophyseal nonapeptide hormone oxytocin (OT), the first peptide hormone to have its structure determined [1], plays an important role in social behavior across a wide variety of species [2, 3]. The word 'oxytocin' was coined from the Greek words (ω k ν ξ, τ o k ox ξ) meaning 'quick birth' after its uterine-contracting properties were discovered by Dale [4]. OT's repertoire has expanded to maintain a central role in more complicated aspects of reproductive behavior. For these reasons, it is called the great facilitator of life [5] (**Figure 1**).

OT is synthesized at the paraventricular (PVN), supraoptic nuclei (SON), and intermediate accessory nuclei of the hypothalamus and transported through the axons of these cells to the posterior pituitary gland [6]. From the posterior pituitary, OT reaches the general blood circulation. It is also produced by different peripheral tissues, such as skin, placenta, ovary, testis, thymus, pancreas, adipocytes, kidney, heart, and blood vessels [7]. OT acts as a hormone in the peripheral circulation and as a neurotransmitter/neuromodulator in the central nervous system [8].

The neurohormone OT is an effective stimulant of the uterine contraction and is used primarily to induce or reinforce labor in obstetrics [9]. OT facilitates the expulsion of milk from the mammary gland during nursing. The release of OT from the posterior pituitary is stimulated by tactile sensory inputs from the nipple. Milk-ejection is the only physiological function known to absolutely require OT [10]. For both men and women, OT is released during sexual stimulation and orgasm, may reduce urine volume and induce natriuresis through co-activation of vasopressin receptors, and is involved in the modulation and regulation of the hypothalamic–pituitary–adrenal (HPA) axis [11]. Moreover, OT plays a role in the

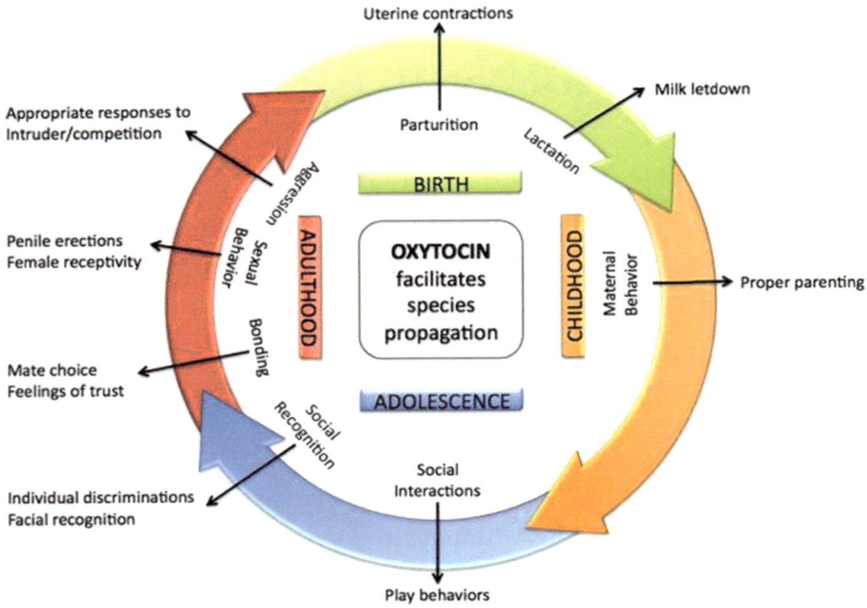

Figure 1.
A simple cycle of life illustrates numerous points at which OT may affect behaviors and physiology to facilitate the propagation of the species [5].

endocrine and paracrine activities such as various sexual and maternal behaviors, social recognition, aggression, neuromodulation, cognition, and tolerance development; however, the mechanism is still unclear [2, 12, 13].

The central neuropeptidergic effect of OT has continued to be studied in the social behavior of various species (in humans and animal models) to date. Nagasawa *et al*. summarized the behavioral and physiological oxytocin-induced effects with the title of "summary of the role of the oxytocin system in reciprocal communication" in **Figure 2** [14].

According to the figure, the central OT secretion is stimulated by multiple sensory signals in mammals. Increased OT release is important in the development of physiology and behavioral functions, and also causes a decrease in pain and stress.

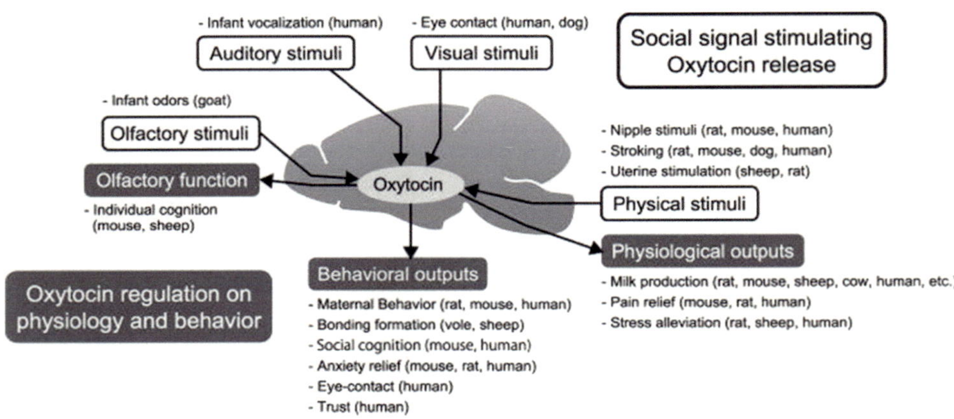

Figure 2.
"Summary of the role of the oxytocin system in reciprocal communication" Nagasawa et al. [14].

2. Chemical properties of oxytocin

Oxytocin (seq;CYIQNCPLG), a neurohypophysial peptide hormone, consists of nine amino acids (H-Cys(1)-Tyr-Ile-Gln-Asn-Cys(1)-Pro-Leu-Gly-NH2) linked with a [1-6] disulfide bond and a semi-flexible carboxy amidation tail [15] (**Figure 3**). This results in a peptide constituted of a rigid N-terminal cyclic 6-residue ring structure and a flexible COOH-terminal alpha amidated three-residue tail [5].

Biological description of IUPAC (International Union of Pure and Applied Chemistry);

H—Cys—Tyr—Ile—Gln—Asn—Cys—Pro—Leu—Gly—NH_2

L-cysteinyl-L-tyrosyl-L-isoleucyl-L-glutaminyl-L-asparagyl-L-cysteinyl-L-prolyl-L-leucyl-glycinamide (1->6)-disulfide [15].

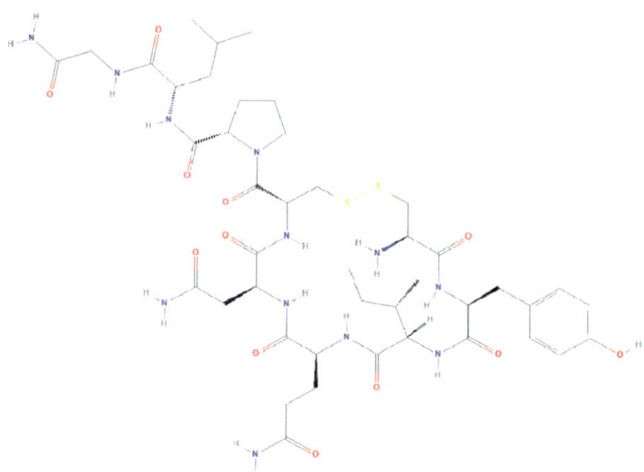

Figure 3.
Chemical structure depiction of oxytocin (OT). Molecular formula: $C_{43}H_{66}N_{12}O_{12}S_2$/Molecular weight: 1007.2 g/mol [15].

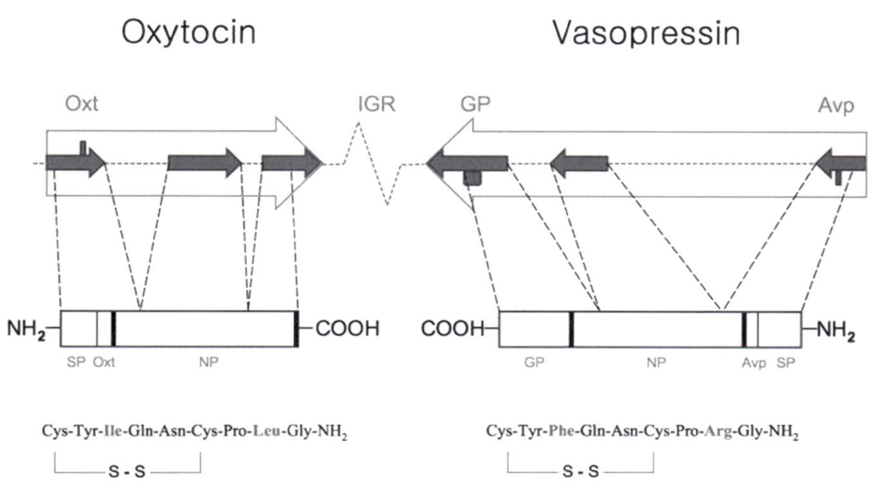

Figure 4.
"Schematic diagram of the oxytocin (OT) and vasopressin (AVP) genes (large arrows), preprohormones (boxes), and neuropeptides (bottom)" [16].

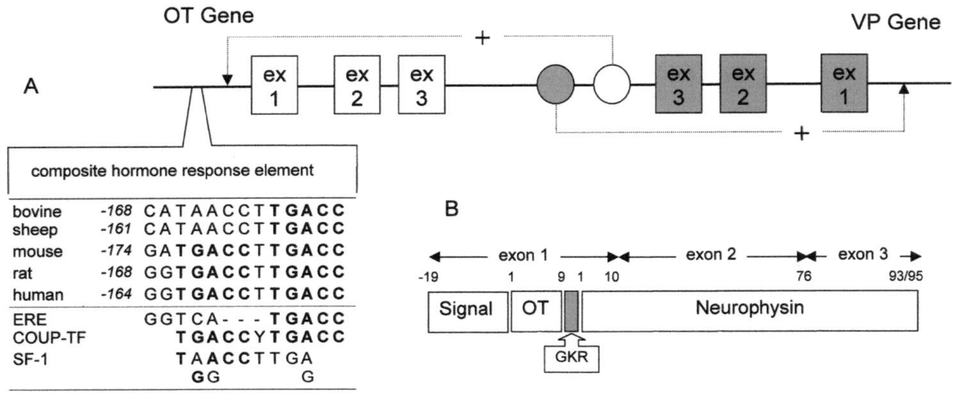

Figure 5.
"Organization of the oxytocin (OT) and vasopressin (VP) gene structure including a schematic depiction of the putative cell-specific enhancers (open circle, enhancer of OT gene; shaded circle, enhancer of VP gene)" [9].

The structure of OT is very similar to another nonapeptide, entitled vasopressin (AVP/arginine vasopressin), which differs from OT by only two amino acids in positions 3 and 8 (**Figure 4**) [16], (**Figure 5**) [9]. OT and AVP genes in the mouse, rat, and human genomes are located on the same chromosome separated by a short (3.5–12 kbp) intergenic region but are in opposite transcriptional orientations [17–20]. They are synthesized in the brain's hypothalamic paraventricular and supraoptic nuclei [21].

3. Oxytocin receptor, cellular actions, and signaling

OT is currently known to have only one receptor (OTR/oxytocin receptor), which forms together with the related V1a, V1b, and V2 vasopressin receptor subtypes a subfamily of the large G protein-coupled receptor (GPCR) superfamily, one of the most abundant protein classes in the mammalian genome [16, 22]. OT shows its biological activity through the GPCR, which is widely expressed throughout the body, including the central and peripheral nervous systems. Heterotrimeric G-proteins are composed of α, β, and γ subunits [23]. These receptors are characterized by seven putative transmembrane domains, three extracellular, and three intracellular loops (**Figure 6**) [9, 22, 24].

The group of OT and vasopressin receptors is well suited for receptor structure–function analysis, because it comprises four related receptors that bind, with varying degrees of specificity, the two closely related peptide ligands, OT and vasopressin [25].

OTR can be coupled to different G proteins, leading to different intracellular pathways. It is possible that these various signaling pathways are differentially expressed in neuronal versus peripheral tissues [26].

The quality of specific acute or long-term neuronal effects of OT is dependent on the regional and subcellular presence of OTR, the characteristics of OT-OTR binding, and subsequent activation of intraneuronal signaling cascades. In addition, the formation of OTR homodimers or heterodimers with other receptors is likely to influence OTR affinity and downstream signaling [23]. The classical signaling pathway associated with the OTR involves a phospholipase C-mediated increase in phosphoinositide hydrolysis, activation of protein kinase C, and a rise in intracellular calcium [27, 28]. The proliferative effects of OT are mediated primarily by the activation of the MAP kinase pathway, involving different G protein-linked pathways as well as receptor tyrosine kinase transactivation [29].

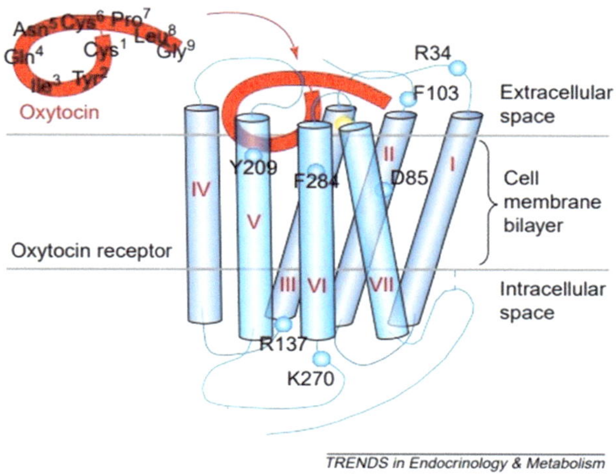

Figure 6.
"Schematic model of the structure of the OT receptor and its interaction with the ligand" (Zingg HH and Laporte SA, 2003) [22].

OT-induced Ca2 influx also seems to play a role in neuronal OT responses. On a cellular level, the OTR activates numerous Ca2-related and MAPK-related signaling cascades in a variety of cell types [23].

Given the multiple signaling pathways in which OTR binds, the development of pathway-specific ligands will be important in elucidating the different OTR-linked pathways, as well as developing more specific agonists and antagonists for future therapeutic applications.

4. Neuroprotective effects of oxytocin hormone

In mammals, increasing brain OT levels promotes attachment and attachment behavior, facilitates parental behavior, social recognition, and memory between relatives, and establishes emotional bonds between animals and caregivers [11, 30–32]. In humans, it has been also shown to increase trust and generosity, strengthen emotional and cognitive empathy, and reduce social-anxiety and fear-related behavior [33, 34]. In line with these findings, impaired social behavior profiles have been associated with reduced central endogenous OTergic activity. Depletion of OTergic signaling through genetic change of the OT gene or receptor has caused convincing social deficiencies, social amnesia, malfunctions in breastfeeding and maternal nutrition, and decreased infant ultrasonic sounds in response to social isolation, but normal birth and sexual behavior [35–37].

Abnormal brain development, during embryogenesis, fetal development, or early postnatal periods, can generate cognitive dysfunction as well as neurological, emotional, and behavioral disorders. Disturbed brain OTergic signaling has been implicated in several psychiatric disorders where social dysfunction is a core symptom (autism spectrum disorder, social anxiety, borderline personality disorder, addiction, and schizophrenia) [31, 37, 38].

There are several animal studies in the literature showing neuroprotective effects of OT. These neuroprotective effects of OT hormone include social neuroprotection, oxygen–glucose deprivation resistance, immune system modulation, anti-apoptotic, anti-inflammatory, and antioxidative functions [38, 39].

Due to the therapeutic properties and health benefits of OT, it can be thought that OT and OT-like molecules are a part of 'natural medicine' that can both prevent and treat diseases and affect the course of many diseases [20].

Understanding the complex actions of OT requires awareness that OT regulates not only the brain and reproductive system but also the immune and autonomic nervous systems. For example, evidence supporting the coordinated effects of acetylcholine (the neurotransmitter in the preganglionic sympathetic and parasympathetic neurons) and OT regulate the autonomic nervous system [40].

The therapeutic effects of the OT hormone have been studied in a variety of pathological conditions, both *in vitro* and *in vivo*.

OT treatment in rats induces several long-lasting anti-stress effects, for example, subchronic OT treatment of males and females rats produces a long-lasting change in spontaneous motor activity, nociception threshold, and weight gain [41].

In many studies, the antiepileptic properties of OT have been emphasized which have positive effects on neurobehavioral pathologies such as autism and psychosis, and it has been shown that it has healing effects on these diseases with its anti-inflammatory and antioxidant properties [42].

It has been revealed that OT modulates the immune and anti-inflammatory response thus reducing inflammatory cytokines production (TNFα; tumor necrosis factor-alpha; is a multifunctional cytokine and IL-6 (interleukin 6)); added to its remarkable anabolic properties on many peripheral organs and on the immune system development [38, 43, 44].

Studies demonstrate the therapeutic effects of both melatonin and OT on critical disease polyneuropathy (CIP) are remarkable. These effects appear to be associated with suppression of cytokine production and improvement in antioxidant capacity [45].

4.1 Vincristine-induced neuropathy

In a study, scientists evaluated the therapeutic potential of OT and liraglutide (LIR), which is a long-acting human glucagon-like peptide-1 (GLP-1) analog, in a rat model of vincristine-induced neuropathy [46]. Vincristine (VCR) is a vinca alkaloid, is known to cause various neurological dysfunctions, antitumoral, and the most neurotoxic agent and it has been used for the treatment of numerous tumors [47, 48]. GLP-1 is a polypeptide hormone composed of 30 amino acids, which is mainly secreted from intestinal L cells in response to nutrient ingestion [49]. Recent studies have indicated that GLP-1 analogs may have therapeutic effects against central and peripheral degenerative changes in animal models of neurodegenerative diseases [50]. GLP-1 exerts its neurotrophic effects through GLP-1 receptors (GLP-1Rs), which are detected particularly on neurons throughout the central and peripheral nervous system [51]. Histological and biochemical findings of the study revealed that both OT and liraglutide significantly prevented neuronal damage by suppressing lipid peroxidation and inducing NGF (nerve growth factor) expression in VCR-received rats [46].

4.2 Cisplatin-induced cytotoxicity

Platinum drugs are compounds containing metal ions that form binding sites for proteins, nucleic acids, and other cellular molecules. This property is largely responsible for the biological activity of drugs as well as their toxicity [52]. Peripheral neurotoxicity is the dose-limiting factor for clinical use of platinum derivatives, a class of anticancer drugs that includes cisplatin, induce decreased neural transmission rate, loss of vibration and position senses, tingling paresthesia, dysesthesia, loss of tendon reflexes, tremor, ataxia, and muscle weakness [53, 54].

Cisplatin (CP) was the first heavy metal compound to be used as antineoplastic, and since its approval by the FDA in 1978, it is one of the most widely used for the treatment of various solid tumors such as lung, ovary, testis, bladder, head, and neck, and cervical and endometrial cancers [55, 56].

The mechanisms suggested explaining the neurotoxicity of these drugs are dorsal root ganglia alteration, oxidative stress involvement, and mitochondrial dysfunction. These alterations are able to stop DNA replication and cell cycle, inhibit DNA repair mechanisms, and induce cell death through apoptosis [57]. Oxidative stress, DNA damage, and inflammatory cytokines play a major role in the mechanism of cisplatin-induced cytotoxicity. Cisplatin increases the production of free oxygen radicals and decreases the antioxidants, thus resulting in the deterioration of the oxidant/antioxidant balance and accumulation of reactive oxygen radicals (ROS) in tissues [58]. Akman *et al.* clearly demonstrated the protective effect of OT in cisplatin-induced neurotoxicity [12]. The neuroprotective effect seems to be associated with antioxidant (by the suppression of lipid peroxidation and increasing the antioxidative capacity) and anti-inflammatory (by decreasing the plasma TNF-α levels) activity of OT [12]. The imbalance between oxidative and antioxidative mechanisms may play an important role in triggering axonal injury [59]. Axonal transport is important for axonal integrity. Excessive ROS production causes distal axonal degeneration and interruption of axonal transportation. It is demonstrated that OT decreases the free oxygen radicals in the brain membranes, prevents low-density lipoprotein oxidation, and inhibits lipid peroxidation [60, 61]. OT decreases the levels of proinflammatory mediators such as TNF-α, IL-4 (interleukin 4) and 6, macrophage inflammatory proteins 1a and 1b, monocyte chemoattractant protein-1, and vascular endothelial growth factor in lipopolysaccharide-induced inflammatory response and endotoxemia [62].

4.3 Diabetic neuropathy

Present results also demonstrate that OT appears to alleviate the harmful effects of hyperglycemia on peripheral neurons by suppressing inflammation, oxidative stress, and apoptotic pathways [63]. Excessive ROS accumulation leads to an increase in mitochondrial inner membrane permeability. Hyperglycemia also increases oxidative stress and inhibits mitochondrial biogenesis [64]. The depletion of growth factors and the activation of caspase 3 and caspase 8 trigger intrinsic apoptotic cell death in neurons [65, 66].

Diabetic polyneuropathy (DNP) is the most common complication of diabetes with a prevalence of 60–70%. DNP represents a heterogeneous group of syndromes with clinical and subclinical disorders and abnormalities such as distal symmetrical polyneuropathy, mononeuropathy, diabetic amyotrophy, autonomic dysfunction, or cranial neuropathies [67]. Hyperglycemia-induced metabolic changes affect tissues and microvascular systems and lead to ischemic pathological changes in the nerve tissue [68]. Erbas *et al.* assessed the neuroprotective and neurorestorative effects of exogenously administered OT on diabetic neuropathy in rats by electrophysiological, biochemical, histological, and immunohistochemical parameters [63]. They demonstrated the potent anti-oxidant and anti-inflammatory effects of different doses of OT on sepsis-induced neuropathy in rats. According to their EMG (electromyography) findings, OT treatment either rescued and/or restored neuromuscular performance in a dose-dependent manner. Following OT treatments, a significant decrease in MDA (malondialdehyde) levels, and a significant increase in GSH (glutathione) levels were detected. The results showed us OT alleviates the harmful effects of hyperglycemia on peripheral neuronal cells by suppressing inflammation, oxidative and apoptotic pathways [63].

4.4 Rotenone induced Parkinson's disease

The brain is the most complex human organ and is extremely sensitive to the action of external chemicals and/or physical factors during its ontogenesis. Exposure to xenobiotics has raised great concern about the increasing prevalence of neurodevelopmental disorders and the possible unknown developmental neurotoxic effects of certain chemicals and drugs [69, 70].

Rotenone is a commonly used plant-derived pesticide that inhibits mitochondrial complex I of the electron transport chain [71]. Rotenone has been suggested as one of the most important environmental risk factors for Parkinson's Disease (PD) [72, 73]. Clinical and experimental studies have strongly supported that it is not only the SNc (substantia nigra pars compacta) and striatum, but also other regions, such as ventral tegmental area (VTA), have important roles in the pathophysiology of PD [74–76]. Accumulating evidence indicates that OT exerts its cytoprotective effects via anti-oxidative, anti-apoptotic, and anti-inflammatory pathways [44, 77, 78]. In recent years, rotenone-induced PD model in rats is commonly used to study the mechanisms of neuronal degeneration in PD. Erbas *et al.* observed a considerable cytoprotective effect of OT on cell death in dopaminergic neurons due to rotenone toxicity [79]. In the study, immunohistochemical evaluation of the brains showed decreased tyrosine hydroxylase immunoreactivity in saline-treated PD animals whereas OT administration significantly enhanced TH (tyrosine hydroxylase) expression in the striatal neurons. Considering that caspase activities play an important role in rotenone-induced cell death, the results obtained from the study revealed that OT reduces apoptosis by affecting mitochondrial caspase pathways and death signals [79]. *In vivo* and *in vitro* studies demonstrate that OT has a triggering role in cell proliferation and neurogenesis [80, 81].

4.5 Hypoxia

The factors that cause brain damage are varied. These factors include inflammation, birth trauma, tumors, stroke, ischemia, and hypoxia, as well as metabolic and genetic disorders. Hypoxia is the insufficient oxygen supply of the cell. It leads to neurodegeneration by causing mitochondrial dysfunction. Disruption of aerobic respiration mechanism causes different degrees of hypoxia in the tissue. As a result of damage, neurodegeneration, and brain dysfunction accompanied by cognitive impairment are observed [82–84]. Depending on the degree of hypoxia, activation of potassium channels, increase in perivascular PH, elevated blood and tissue concentrations of CO2, variation in intracellular calcium levels may contribute to neurodegeneration [85]. Regardless of neuronal damage, another factor underlying hypoxia-induced neonatal seizures may be a decrease in gamma-aminobutyric acid (GABA) activity [42, 86]. The cerebral cortex, hippocampus, striatum, and cerebellum have been shown to be the primary areas that are significantly affected by hypoxia and these regions have been associated with the resultant long-term cognitive problems in animal models [87]. In 2018, Panaitescu *et al.* reported that OT showed hippocampal neuroprotective effects and reduced the number of cumulative seizures in hypoxia-induced rats [88]. OT suppresses inflammation in the central nervous system and has another vital role that concerns GABA (gamma-aminobutyric acid; a neurotransmitter in the brain); it alternates the GABAergic neurons from depolarizing to hyperpolarizing in terms of supporting normal anoxia associated with labor and delivery [88–90]. In a study, results showed that OT treatment given in the acute period of hypoxia had ameliorative effects on PTZ (pentylenetetrazol; a GABA(A) receptor antagonist)-induced convulsions in the long term. Also, it was observed significantly decreased TNF-α level in both of the hypoxia groups that were given OT treatment [91]. Possible mechanisms of this effect were hormone suppresses inflammation and reduces hippocampal gliosis, and anticonvulsant effect by increasing GABAergic activity. That conclusion was exemplified by the significantly decreased TNF-α level in both of the hypoxia groups that were given OT treatment. Brain inflammation caused by LPS (lipopolysaccharide) is characterized by neuronal loss and microglial activation. Findings have demonstrated that OT suppressed lipopolysaccharide-induced microglial activation [91, 92]. Studies also have shown that OT reduces the release of cytokines such as TNF-α, IL-6, IL-1β (interleukin 1 beta), IFN-γ (interferon-gamma) by suppressing inflammation [93].

4.6 Stroke

Stroke is a sudden decrease or cessation of blood flow to the brain. It can occur when one of the brain vessels ruptures and blood bleeds into the brain tissue or brain membranes. This is known as "brain hemorrhage". Depending on the affected brain region, speech, muscle strength, coordination-balance, vision, or memory loss occur. Technical advances in neuroimaging and neuropathology have facilitated the understanding of ischemia, infarction, and hemorrhage in the brain [94]. Neuronal injury in stroke is caused by different mechanisms, including excitotoxicity, inflammation, oxidative stress, and apoptosis [95].

Cerebral ischemia induces microglial activation by a strong inflammatory reaction with peripheral leukocyte influx into the cerebral parenchyma. Interruption of cerebral blood flow causes necrotic neuron death by affecting energy metabolism. In addition, different immune responses occur and inflammatory cell activation develops. Inflammatory cells can release a variety of cytotoxic agents including more cytokines, matrix metalloproteinases (MMPs), nitric oxide (NO), and more ROS (**Figure 7**) [95, 96].

One of the dramatic events during ischemia is the increase in intracellular calcium (Ca + 2), which leads to the activation of calpain proteases [97]. A study shows that calpain-1 increases reactive oxygen species levels and inflammatory cytokines [98]. Increased oxidative stress followed by calcium influx, mitochondrial dysfunction, and the loss of cytoskeletal proteins are phenotypes commonly observed in Alzheimer, Huntington, and Parkinson's diseases, as well as amyotrophic lateral sclerosis, stroke, ischemia, spinal cord injury, and TBI (traumatic brain injury) [99].

Neuroprotective effects of OT and the underlying molecular mechanisms are under discussion after different ischemia–reperfusion models [100, 101]. Jankowski *et al* reported that treatment with OT after cardiac ischemic induction in rats can reduce myocardial infarct size and improve heart function [102]. In a study, Etehadi *et al* showed a significant decrease in calpain-1 expression after OT administration in the tMCAO (transient middle cerebral artery occlusion) model. This refers to the neuroprotective role of OT, which could result in the inhibition of calpain [38]. Overall, these findings will add to our knowledge of the positive effects of OT on the outcomes of stroke.

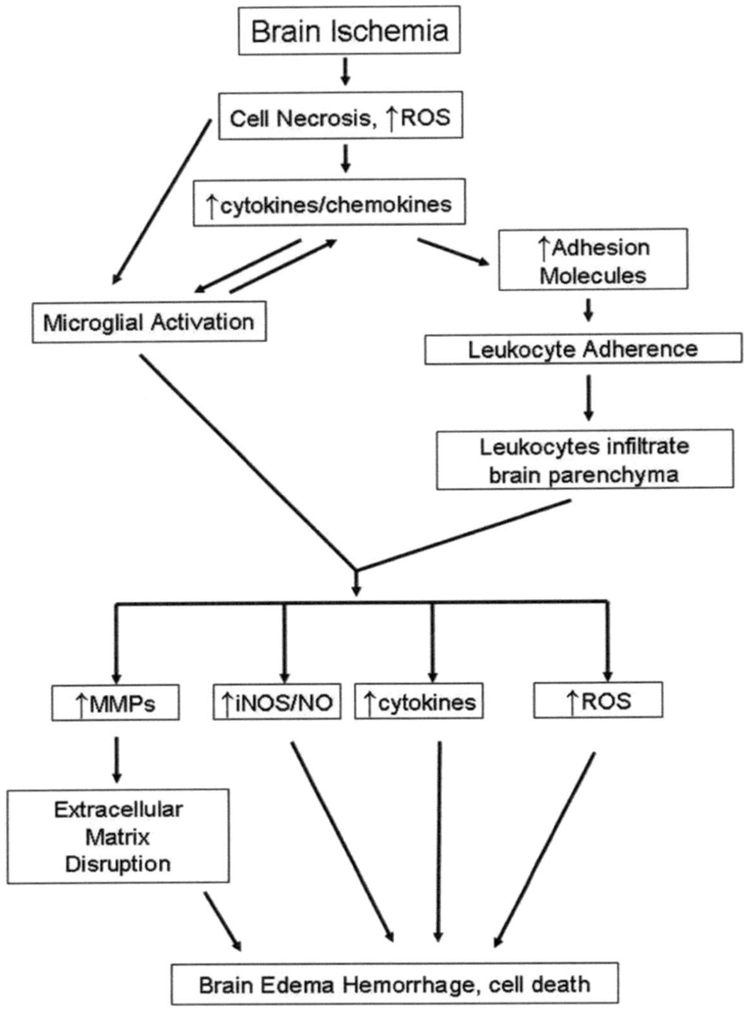

Figure 7.
"Brain ischemia triggers inflammatory responses due to the presence of necrotic cells, generation of reactive oxygen species (ROS), and production of inflammatory cytokines even within neurons" (Wang Q et al. 2007) [95].

5. Summary and discussion

The effect of oxytocin as a neuromodulator is a subject that has been studied in many different ways. It effectively provides nerve regeneration in nerve damage is a known issue. In addition, its anti-epileptic attack or reducing attack power effect in epilepsy models has also been shown in some studies. It plays an important role in the regulation of spinal autonomic functions. Although it regulates urination reflex and uterine motility, it can increase heart rate and renal sympathetic activity. Considering the positive effects of OT on the brain, reproductive system, immune and autonomic nervous system it shows promise as future treatment agents on the spectrum of anxiety, autism, personality disorders, and neurodegenerative disorders. Studies reveal that oxytocin shows its cytoprotective effects through its anti-inflammatory, anti-apoptotic and antioxidant properties. In chronic inflammation, immune cells constantly attack healthy tissues, resulting in conditions such as obesity, cancer, diabetes, heart disease, autoimmune diseases, Alzheimer's, and some other diseases. Increasing the effectiveness of anti-inflammatory agents such as OT will improve the quality of life by changing the course of many diseases.

Author details

Oytun Erbaş[1,2]* and İlknur Altuntaş[1,2]*

1 ERBAS Institute of Experimental Medicine, Illinois, USA

2 ERBAS Institute of Experimental Medicine, Gebze, Turkey

*Address all correspondence to: oytunerbas@yahoo.com
and ilknuraltuntas@gmail.com

References

[1] Du Vigneaud V, Ressler C, Trippett S. The sequence of amino acids in oxytocin, with a proposal for the structure of oxytocin. J Biol Chem. 1953;205: 949-957.

[2] Bartz JA, Zaki J, Bolger N, Ochsner KN. Social effects of oxytocin in humans: context and person matter. Trends Cogn Sci. 2011;15: 301-309.

[3] Ebert A, Brüne M. Oxytocin and Social Cognition. Curr Top Behav Neurosci. 2018;35: 375-388.

[4] Dale HH. On some physiological actions of ergot. The Journal of Physiology. 1906. pp. 163-206.

[5] Lee H-J, Macbeth AH, Pagani JH, Young WS 3rd. Oxytocin: the great facilitator of life. Prog Neurobiol. 2009;88: 127-151.

[6] Quintana DS, Guastella AJ. An Allostatic Theory of Oxytocin. Trends Cogn Sci. 2020;24: 515-528.

[7] Hortu I, Ozceltik G, Ergenoglu AM, Yigitturk G, Atasoy O, Erbas O. Protective effect of oxytocin on a methotrexate-induced ovarian toxicity model. Arch Gynecol Obstet. 2020;301: 1317-1324.

[8] Churchland PS, Winkielman P. Modulating social behavior with oxytocin: how does it work? What does it mean? Horm Behav. 2012;61: 392-399.

[9] Gimpl G, Fahrenholz F. The oxytocin receptor system: structure, function, and regulation. Physiol Rev. 2001;81: 629-683.

[10] Macuhová J, Tancin V, Bruckmaier RM. Effects of oxytocin administration on oxytocin release and milk ejection. J Dairy Sci. 2004;87: 1236-1244.

[11] Insel TR. The Challenge of Translation in Social Neuroscience: A Review of Oxytocin, Vasopressin, and Affiliative Behavior. Neuron. 2010. pp. 768-779.

[12] Akman T, Akman L, Erbas O, Terek MC, Taskiran D, Ozsaran A. The preventive effect of oxytocin to Cisplatin-induced neurotoxicity: an experimental rat model. Biomed Res Int. 2015;2015: 167235.

[13] Heinrichs M, von Dawans B, Domes G. Oxytocin, vasopressin, and human social behavior. Front Neuroendocrinol. 2009;30: 548-557.

[14] Nagasawa M, Okabe S, Mogi K, Kikusui T. Oxytocin and mutual communication in mother-infant bonding. Front Hum Neurosci. 2012.

[15] Website. [cited 14 Jan 2021]. Available: PubChem [Internet]. Bethesda (MD): National Library of Medicine (US), National Center for Biotechnology Information; 2004-. PubChem Compound Summary for CID 439302, Oxytocin; [cited 2021 Jan. 9]. Available from: https://pubchem.ncbi.nlm.nih.gov/compound/Oxytocin

[16] Caldwell HK, Lee H-J, Macbeth AH, Young WS 3rd. Vasopressin: behavioral roles of an "original" neuropeptide. Prog Neurobiol. 2008;84: 1-24.

[17] Gainer H. Cell-specific gene expression in oxytocin and vasopressin magnocellular neurons. Adv Exp Med Biol. 1998;449: 15-27.

[18] Farina-Lipari E, Valentino B. Immunohistochemical research on vasopressin in the accessory hypothalamic nuclei. Ital J Anat Embryol. 1993;98: 207-214.

[19] Farina Lipari E, Valentino B, Lipari D. Immunohistochemical

research on oxytocin in the hypothalamic accessory nuclei. Ital J Anat Embryol. 1995;100: 189-193.

[20] Carter CS, Sue Carter C, Kenkel WM, MacLean EL, Wilson SR, Perkeybile AM, et al. Is Oxytocin "Nature's Medicine"? Pharmacological Reviews. 2020. pp. 829-861.

[21] Keverne EB, Curley JP. Vasopressin, oxytocin and social behaviour. Curr Opin Neurobiol. 2004;14: 777-783.

[22] Zingg HH, Laporte SA. The oxytocin receptor. Trends Endocrinol Metab. 2003;14: 222-227.

[23] Jurek B, Neumann ID. The Oxytocin Receptor: From Intracellular Signaling to Behavior. Physiol Rev. 2018;98: 1805-1908.

[24] Breton C, Chellil H, Kabbaj-Benmansour M, Carnazzi E, Seyer R, Phalipou S, et al. Direct Identification of Human Oxytocin Receptor-binding Domains Using a Photoactivatable Cyclic Peptide Antagonist. Journal of Biological Chemistry. 2001. pp. 26931-26941.

[25] Postina R, Kojro E, Fahrenholz F. Separate Agonist and Peptide Antagonist Binding Sites of the Oxytocin Receptor Defined by Their Transfer into the V2Vasopressin Receptor. Journal of Biological Chemistry. 1996. pp. 31593-31601.

[26] Stoop R. Neuromodulation by Oxytocin and Vasopressin. Neuron. 2012. pp. 142-159.

[27] Ku CY, Qian A, Wen Y, Anwer K, Sanborn BM. Oxytocin stimulates myometrial guanosine triphosphatase and phospholipase-C activities via coupling to G alpha q/11. Endocrinology. 1995. pp. 1509-1515.

[28] Sanborn BM, Dodge K, Monga M, Qian A, Wang W, Yue C. Molecular mechanisms regulating the effects of oxytocin on myometrial intracellular calcium. Adv Exp Med Biol. 1998;449: 277-286.

[29] Wrzal PK, Goupil E, Laporte SA, Hébert TE, Zingg HH. Functional interactions between the oxytocin receptor and the β2-adrenergic receptor: implications for ERK1/2 activation in human myometrial cells. Cell Signal. 2012;24: 333-341.

[30] Neumann ID, Landgraf R. Balance of brain oxytocin and vasopressin: implications for anxiety, depression, and social behaviors. Trends Neurosci. 2012;35: 649-659.

[31] Bielsky IF, Young LJ. Oxytocin, vasopressin, and social recognition in mammals. Peptides. 2004;25: 1565-1574.

[32] Ferguson JN, Matthew Aldag J, Insel TR, Young LJ. Oxytocin in the Medial Amygdala is Essential for Social Recognition in the Mouse. J Neurosci. 2001. pp. 8278-8285.

[33] Barraza JA, Zak PJ. Empathy toward strangers triggers oxytocin release and subsequent generosity. Ann N Y Acad Sci. 2009;1167: 182-189.

[34] Neumann ID. Oxytocin: the neuropeptide of love reveals some of its secrets. Cell Metab. 2007;5: 231-233.

[35] Ferguson JN, Young LJ, Hearn EF, Matzuk MM, Insel TR, Winslow JT. Social amnesia in mice lacking the oxytocin gene. Nat Genet. 2000;25: 284-288.

[36] Winslow JT, Insel TR. The social deficits of the oxytocin knockout mouse. Neuropeptides. 2002;36: 221-229.

[37] Witt DM, Winslow JT, Insel TR. Enhanced social interactions in rats following chronic, centrally infused

oxytocin. Pharmacol Biochem Behav. 1992;43: 855-861.

[38] Etehadi Moghadam S, Azami Tameh A, Vahidinia Z, Atlasi MA, Hassani Bafrani H, Naderian H. Neuroprotective Effects of Oxytocin Hormone after an Experimental Stroke Model and the Possible Role of Calpain-1. J Stroke Cerebrovasc Dis. 2018;27: 724-732.

[39] Vargas-Martínez F, Uvnäs-Moberg K, Petersson M, Olausson HA, Jiménez-Estrada I. Neuropeptides as neuroprotective agents: Oxytocin a forefront developmental player in the mammalian brain. Prog Neurobiol. 2014;123: 37-78.

[40] Freeman SM, Young LJ. Comparative Perspectives on Oxytocin and Vasopressin Receptor Research in Rodents and Primates: Translational Implications. J Neuroendocrinol. 2016;28.

[41] Pedersen CA. Oxytocin control of maternal behavior. Regulation by sex steroids and offspring stimuli. Ann N Y Acad Sci. 1997;807: 126-145.

[42] Kaneko Y, Pappas C, Tajiri N, Borlongan CV. Oxytocin modulates GABAR subunits to confer neuroprotection in stroke in vitro. Sci Rep. 2016;6: 35659.

[43] Tamma R, Colaianni G, Zhu L-L, DiBenedetto A, Greco G, Montemurro G, et al. Oxytocin is an anabolic bone hormone. Proc Natl Acad Sci U S A. 2009;106: 7149-7154.

[44] Rashed LA, Hashem RM, Soliman HM. Oxytocin inhibits NADPH oxidase and P38 MAPK in cisplatin-induced nephrotoxicity. Biomed Pharmacother. 2011;65: 474-480.

[45] Erbaş O, Ergenoglu AM, Akdemir A, Yeniel AÖ, Taskiran D. Comparison of melatonin and oxytocin in the prevention of critical illness polyneuropathy in rats with experimentally induced sepsis. J Surg Res. 2013;183: 313-320.

[46] Erdoğan MA, Taşkıran E, Yiğittürk G, Erbaş O, Taşkıran D. The investigation of therapeutic potential of oxytocin and liraglutide on vincristine-induced neuropathy in rats. J Biochem Mol Toxicol. 2020;34: e22415.

[47] Li G-Z, Hu Y-H, Li D-Y, Zhang Y, Guo H-L, Li Y-M, et al. Vincristine-induced peripheral neuropathy: A mini-review. Neurotoxicology. 2020;81: 161-171.

[48] Yang L, Yu L, Chen X, Hu Y, Wang B. Clinical Analysis of Adverse Drug Reactions between Vincristine and Triazoles in Children with Acute Lymphoblastic Leukemia. Med Sci Monit. 2015;21: 1656-1661.

[49] Drucker DJ, Habener JF, Holst JJ. Discovery, characterization, and clinical development of the glucagon-like peptides. J Clin Invest. 2017;127: 4217-4227.

[50] Chen S, Liu A-R, An F-M, Yao W-B, Gao X-D. Amelioration of neurodegenerative changes in cellular and rat models of diabetes-related Alzheimer's disease by exendin-4. Age. 2012;34: 1211-1224.

[51] Perry T, Lahiri DK, Chen D, Zhou J, Shaw KTY, Egan JM, et al. A novel neurotrophic property of glucagon-like peptide 1: a promoter of nerve growth factor-mediated differentiation in PC12 cells. J Pharmacol Exp Ther. 2002;300: 958-966.

[52] McWhinney SR, Goldberg RM, McLeod HL. Platinum neurotoxicity pharmacogenetics. Mol Cancer Ther. 2009;8: 10-16.

[53] Chiorazzi A, Semperboni S, Marmiroli P. Current View in Platinum Drug Mechanisms of Peripheral Neurotoxicity. Toxics. 2015;3: 304-321.

[54] Pace A, Giannarelli D, Galiè E, Savarese A, Carpano S, Della Giulia M, et al. Vitamin E neuroprotection for cisplatin neuropathy: a randomized, placebo-controlled trial. Neurology. 2010;74: 762-766.

[55] Santos NAGD, Ferreira RS, Santos ACD. Overview of cisplatin-induced neurotoxicity and ototoxicity, and the protective agents. Food Chem Toxicol. 2020;136: 111079.

[56] Cepeda V, Fuertes MA, Castilla J, Alonso C, Quevedo C, Pérez JM. Biochemical mechanisms of cisplatin cytotoxicity. Anticancer Agents Med Chem. 2007;7: 3-18.

[57] Ciarimboli G. Membrane transporters as mediators of Cisplatin effects and side effects. Scientifica. 2012;2012: 473829.

[58] Kawai Y, Nakao T, Kunimura N, Kohda Y, Gemba M. Relationship of intracellular calcium and oxygen radicals to Cisplatin-related renal cell injury. J Pharmacol Sci. 2006;100: 65-72.

[59] Bordt EA, Polster BM. NADPH oxidase- and mitochondria-derived reactive oxygen species in proinflammatory microglial activation: a bipartisan affair? Free Radic Biol Med. 2014;76: 34-46.

[60] Moosmann B, Behl C. Secretory peptide hormones are biochemical antioxidants: structure-activity relationship. Mol Pharmacol. 2002;61: 260-268.

[61] Evans MD, Dizdaroglu M, Cooke MS. Oxidative DNA damage and disease: induction, repair and significance. Mutat Res. 2004;567: 1-61.

[62] Clodi M, Vila G, Geyeregger R, Riedl M, Stulnig TM, Struck J, et al. Oxytocin alleviates the neuroendocrine and cytokine response to bacterial endotoxin in healthy men. Am J Physiol Endocrinol Metab. 2008;295: E686–E691.

[63] Erbas O, Taşkıran D, Oltulu F, Yavaşoğlu A, Bora S, Bilge O, et al. Oxytocin provides protection against diabetic polyneuropathy in rats. Neurol Res. 2017;39: 45-53.

[64] Kaludercic N, Di Lisa F. Mitochondrial ROS Formation in the Pathogenesis of Diabetic Cardiomyopathy. Frontiers in Cardiovascular Medicine. 2020.

[65] Redza-Dutordoir M, Averill-Bates DA. Activation of apoptosis signalling pathways by reactive oxygen species. Biochim Biophys Acta. 2016;1863: 2977-2992.

[66] Hollville E, Romero SE, Deshmukh M. Apoptotic cell death regulation in neurons. FEBS J. 2019;286: 3276-3298.

[67] Dyck PJ, Giannini C. Pathologic alterations in the diabetic neuropathies of humans: a review. J Neuropathol Exp Neurol. 1996;55: 1181-1193.

[68] Güemes A, Georgiou P. Review of the role of the nervous system in glucose homoeostasis and future perspectives towards the management of diabetes. Bioelectron Med. 2018;4: 9.

[69] Grandjean P, Landrigan PJ. Developmental neurotoxicity of industrial chemicals. The Lancet. 2006. pp. 2167-2178.

[70] Schettler T. Toxic threats to neurologic development of children. Environmental Health Perspectives. 2001. pp. 813-816.

[71] Saravanan KS, Sindhu KM, Mohanakumar KP. Acute intranigral infusion of rotenone in rats causes progressive biochemical lesions in the striatum similar to Parkinson's disease. Brain Res. 2005;1049: 147-155.

[72] Perier C, Bové J, Vila M, Przedborski S. The rotenone model of Parkinson's disease. Trends Neurosci. 2003;26: 345-346.

[73] Sherer TB, Betarbet R, Testa CM, Seo BB, Richardson JR, Kim JH, et al. Mechanism of Toxicity in Rotenone Models of Parkinson's Disease. J Neurosci. 2003. pp. 10756-10764.

[74] German DC, Manaye K, Smith WK, Woodward DJ, Saper CB. Midbrain dopaminergic cell loss in Parkinson's disease: computer visualization. Ann Neurol. 1989;26: 507-514.

[75] Vernier P, Moret F, Callier S, Snapyan M, Wersinger C, Sidhu A. The degeneration of dopamine neurons in Parkinson's disease: insights from embryology and evolution of the mesostriatocortical system. Ann N Y Acad Sci. 2004;1035: 231-249.

[76] Lim S-Y, Fox SH, Lang AE. Overview of the extranigral aspects of Parkinson disease. Arch Neurol. 2009;66: 167-172.

[77] Petersson M, Lagumdzija A, Stark A, Bucht E. Oxytocin stimulates proliferation of human osteoblast-like cells. Peptides. 2002;23: 1121-1126.

[78] Jankowski M, Broderick TL, Gutkowska J. The Role of Oxytocin in Cardiovascular Protection. Frontiers in Psychology. 2020.

[79] Erbaş O, Oltulu F, Taşkiran D. Amelioration of rotenone-induced dopaminergic cell death in the striatum by oxytocin treatment. Peptides. 2012;38: 312-317.

[80] Bakos J, Strbak V, Ratulovska N, Bacova Z. Effect of oxytocin on neuroblastoma cell viability and growth. Cell Mol Neurobiol. 2012;32: 891-896.

[81] Leuner B, Caponiti JM, Gould E. Oxytocin stimulates adult neurogenesis even under conditions of stress and elevated glucocorticoids. Hippocampus. 2012;22: 861-868.

[82] Gonzalez FF, Ferriero DM. Therapeutics for neonatal brain injury. Pharmacol Ther. 2008;120: 43-53.

[83] Gressens P, Luton D. Fetal MRI: obstetrical and neurological perspectives. Pediatr Radiol. 2004;34: 682-684.

[84] Byeon JH, Kim G-H, Kim JY, Sun W, Kim H, Eun B-L. Cognitive Dysfunction and Hippocampal Damage Induced by Hypoxic-Ischemic Brain Injury and Prolonged Febrile Convulsions in Immature Rats. J Korean Neurosurg Soc. 2015. p. 22.

[85] Faraci FM, Taugher RJ, Lynch C, Fan R, Gupta S, Wemmie JA. Acid-Sensing Ion Channels. Circ Res. 2019. pp. 907-920.

[86] Yoon S, Kim Y-K. The Role of the Oxytocin System in Anxiety Disorders. Adv Exp Med Biol. 2020. pp. 103-120.

[87] Pozdnyakova N. Consequences of perinatal hypoxia in developing brain: Changes in GABA transporter functioning in cortical, hippocampal and thalamic rat nerve terminals. Int J Dev Neurosci. 2017;63: 1-7.

[88] Panaitescu A. Oxytocin Reduces Seizure Burden and Hippocampal Injury in a Rat Model of Perinatal Asphyxia. Acta Endocrinologica (Bucharest). 2018. pp. 315-319.

[89] Khazipov R, Tyzio R, Ben-Ari Y. Effects of oxytocin on GABA signalling

in the foetal brain during delivery. Prog Brain Res. 2008;170: 243-257.

[90] Xu S, Qin B, Shi A, Zhao J, Guo X, Dong L. Oxytocin inhibited stress induced visceral hypersensitivity, enteric glial cells activation, and release of proinflammatory cytokines in maternal separated rats. Eur J Pharmacol. 2018. pp. 578-584.

[91] Sünnetçi E, Solmaz V, Erbaş O. Chronic Oxytocin treatment has long lasting therapeutic potential in a rat model of neonatal hypercapnic-hypoxia injury, through enhanced GABAergic signaling and by reducing hippocampal gliosis with its anti-inflammatory feature. Peptides. 2021. p. 170398.

[92] Inoue T, Yamakage H, Tanaka M, Kusakabe T, Shimatsu A, Satoh-Asahara N. Oxytocin Suppresses Inflammatory Responses Induced by Lipopolysaccharide through Inhibition of the eIF-2α–ATF4 Pathway in Mouse Microglia. Cells. 2019. p. 527.

[93] Wang S-C, Lin C-C, Chen C-C, Tzeng N-S, Liu Y-P. Effects of Oxytocin on Fear Memory and Neuroinflammation in a Rodent Model of Posttraumatic Stress Disorder. Int J Mol Sci. 2018. p. 3848.

[94] Sacco RL, Kasner SE, Broderick JP, Caplan LR, Connors JJB, Culebras A, et al. An updated definition of stroke for the 21st century: a statement for healthcare professionals from the American Heart Association/American Stroke Association. Stroke. 2013;44: 2064-2089.

[95] Wang Q, Tang XN, Yenari MA. The inflammatory response in stroke. J Neuroimmunol. 2007;184: 53-68.

[96] Emsley HCA, Tyrrell PJ. Inflammation and infection in clinical stroke. J Cereb Blood Flow Metab. 2002;22: 1399-1419.

[97] Neumar RW, Meng FH, Mills AM, Anne Xu Y, Zhang C, Welsh FA, et al. Calpain Activity in the Rat Brain after Transient Forebrain Ischemia. Exp Neurol. 2001. pp. 27-35.

[98] Yamada KH, Kozlowski DA, Seidl SE, Lance S, Wieschhaus AJ, Sundivakkam P, et al. Targeted Gene Inactivation of Calpain-1 Suppresses Cortical Degeneration Due to Traumatic Brain Injury and Neuronal Apoptosis Induced by Oxidative Stress. J Biol Chem. 2012. pp. 13182-13193.

[99] Higgins GC, Beart PM, Shin YS, Chen MJ, Cheung NS, Nagley P. Oxidative stress: emerging mitochondrial and cellular themes and variations in neuronal injury. J Alzheimers Dis. 2010;20 Suppl 2: S453–S473.

[100] Akdemir A, Erbas O, Gode F, Ergenoglu M, Yeniel O, Oltulu F, et al. Protective effect of oxytocin on ovarian ischemia-reperfusion injury in rats. Peptides. 2014;55: 126-130.

[101] Tuğtepe H, Sener G, Biyikli NK, Yüksel M, Cetinel S, Gedik N, et al. The protective effect of oxytocin on renal ischemia/reperfusion injury in rats. Regul Pept. 2007;140: 101-108.

[102] Jankowski M, Bissonauth V, Gao L, Gangal M, Wang D, Danalache B, et al. Anti-inflammatory effect of oxytocin in rat myocardial infarction. Basic Res Cardiol. 2010;105: 205-218.

Chapter 5

Priming the Pathway: Combining Oxytocin and Behavioral Intervention to Improve Outcomes in Autism Spectrum Disorder

Katherine Kuhl Meltzoff Stavropoulos and Elizabeth Baker

Abstract

Autism spectrum disorder (ASD) is a neurodevelopmental disorder characterized by social-communication deficits and the presence of restricted interests and/or repetitive behaviors. There are currently no psychopharmacological agents approved to treat core symptoms of ASD. As such, behavioral interventions are the most effective method for improving symptoms. In the current chapter, we propose that administering the neuropeptide oxytocin in conjunction with evidence-based behavioral interventions may lead to improved outcomes in social-communication for children with ASD. From a mechanistic perspective, we hypothesize that oxytocin may "prime" social reward circuitry in the brain, thereby allowing behavioral interventions designed to increase social motivation/initiation to be more effective. Extant literature related to theories of ASD, oxytocin administration in children with ASD, and behavioral intervention outcomes are reviewed, and considerations for individual characteristics (e.g., genetics, oxytocin availability, age, behavioral profile, etc.) that may affect efficacy are discussed.

Keywords: Autism spectrum disorder (ASD), Social Motivation, Oxytocin, Intervention, Reward, outcomes, neuroscience

1. Introduction

It is estimated that 1 in 59 children in the United States has a diagnosis of Autism Spectrum Disorder (ASD) [1], which is characterized by life-long social communication deficits and the presence of restricted interests and/or repetitive behaviors [2]. Though all individuals with ASD meet common diagnostic criteria, they display a wide spectrum of behavioral manifestations, thus producing a wide array of heterogeneous phenotypes. As such, a multitude of behavioral interventions exist to address common symptoms of ASD, many of which have been tailored to address the heterogeneity of the disorder. Behavioral interventions are currently one of the most effective methods for improving social-communication skills, as no medications have been approved to "treat" social communication behaviors in ASD.

In the current chapter, we propose that administering the neuropeptide oxytocin in conjunction with evidence-based behavioral interventions may lead to improved outcomes in social-communication for children with ASD. Specifically, we propose that oxytocin administration may "prime" social reward circuitry in the brain, allowing behavioral interventions designed to increase social motivation/initiation to be more effective. This theoretical model draws from the following research: (1) the social motivation hypothesis of ASD, (2) animal and human literature related to oxytocin, (3) studies of oxytocin levels in children with ASD, (4) behavioral changes after oxytocin administration in children with ASD, (5) neural changes after oxytocin administration in children with ASD, and (6) neural changes after behavioral interventions in children with ASD.

Subsequent sections will briefly review these research areas. We propose that taken together, the aforementioned literature provides a theoretical basis for combining oxytocin administration with behavioral interventions to improve social-communicative outcomes for children with ASD.

2. Social motivation hypothesis of ASD

The social motivation hypothesis posits that early impairments in social attention (due to social stimuli being less rewarding for individuals with ASD compared to their neurotypical peers) set a series of negative developmental consequences in motion. Initial impairments in social attention--which often manifest as decreased orienting to one's own name, diminished eye contact, and decreased social initiations in early life--lead to fewer opportunities for social learning, which in turn lead to deficits in social communication, social skills, and social-cognitive development [3, 4]. The proposed neural mechanisms underlying the social motivation hypothesis are the reward centers in the brain including the amygdala, ventral striatum, and orbito-frontal cortex [4]. Importantly, social motivation is thought to involve both oxytocin and the dopaminergic reward pathways [5, 6]. Given the hypothesized role of oxytocin in social motivation, it is not surprising that oxytocin has been considered as a potential mechanism for understanding social deficits in ASD--and that oxytocin administration has been considered as a potential therapeutic agent.

3. Oxytocin overview

Oxytocin is a neuropeptide produced in the hypothalamus [7]. Colloquially referred to as the "love hormone," oxytocin has been implicated in the formation of pair bonds in a variety of species, including rats and prairie voles [8–10]. As such, oxytocin has been extensively studied and utilized for its effects on social cognition and prosocial behaviors [11–13]. It has been hypothesized that interactions between oxytocin and the dopaminergic reward system support social affiliative behaviors and social bonds [14]. Further evidence of the connection between oxytocin and the dopamine reward system comes from overlap in locations of receptor binding sites and neuronal fibers [15]. Furthermore, oxytocin cells in the hypothalamus have been found to express dopamine receptors [16]. Importantly for neurodevelopmental disorders such as ASD, oxytocin is developmentally regulated and its receptors are malleable, particularly in response to parent-child interactions [17, 18].

In contrast to other conditions in which both behavioral and medical treatments are supported by empirical evidence, no medication is currently approved to improve core symptoms of ASD. Although two pharmaceutical medications, risperidone and aripiprazole, have been approved by the Federal Drug Administration for use in ASD, they do not address core symptoms. Rather, they have been approved to treat ancillary symptoms of ASD, such as aggression and irritability [19]. Due to the lack of pharmacological interventions to address the core symptoms of ASD, there has been a focus on compounds that directly address social communication symptoms. Given oxytocin's role in prosocial behaviors, exogenous administration of the neuropeptide has been considered as a potential therapeutic agent in ASD.

3.1 Oxytocin levels in ASD

Modahl and colleagues [20, 21] were the first to provide evidence of reduced levels of oxytocin in children with ASD. Specifically, the authors found that compared to their neurotypical peers, oxytocin does not increase prior to the onset of puberty in individuals with ASD. This suggests that oxytocin is less available to individuals with ASD during development [21]. Our understanding of oxytocin in individuals with ASD has since been shaped by research that suggests deficits in oxytocin may reveal the pathogenesis of ASD. No known mechanistic pathway exists to form a substantial link between the neuropeptide and development of ASD, but studies support the idea that lower concentrations of oxytocin are strongly related to social impairments [22].

Early studies of the endocrine system have found that oxytocin release occurs differently in children with ASD compared to their neurotypical peers, suggesting that oxytocin may be disrupted early in development in children with ASD [23]. Oxytocin blood plasma levels increase throughout neurotypical development, while children with ASD exhibit lower levels of plasma oxytocin [24] that are stable over time [21]. Therefore, disruptions of the oxytocin system may possibly occur early in life in individuals with ASD, resulting in cascading consequences.

4. Oxytocin administration in children with ASD

4.1 Behavioral findings

To our knowledge, eight studies have been conducted to measure behavioral results of oxytocin administration for children with ASD [22, 24–33]. Though the current chapter focuses on children, see the meta-analysis by Ooi and colleagues [32] for a review of randomized control trials of oxytocin administration in both children and adults. See **Table 1**.

In 2010, Guastella and colleagues [25] completed a double-blind placebo-controlled study with 16 adolescent boys with ASD (ages 12-19). 45 minutes after oxytocin (or placebo) administration, participants completed the Reading the Mind in the Eyes Task, or RMET [33]. Compared to placebo, oxytocin improved performance on the REMET for 60% of participants. When the authors split REMET items into "easy" and "hard" categories, the effect of oxytocin was particularly significant for "easy" items. This was the first investigation of the results of oxytocin administration to children/adolescents, and suggested that oxytocin improves emotion recognition in a group of males with ASD.

Tachibana and colleagues [26] measured behavioral changes associated with an open label (participants knew they were receiving oxytocin), single arm (no placebo condition) long-term oxytocin administration in 8 boys with ASD (ages 10-14). Participants received intranasal oxytocin twice a day for approximately 7 months. Oxytocin dosage was increased in a stepwise fashion every 2 months (from an initial dose of 8 IU to 24 IU). Outcome measures were scores on the Autism Diagnostic Observation Schedule—Generic (ADOS-G; [34]), Aberrant Behavior Checklist (ABC; [35]), and Child Behavior Checklist (CBCL; [36]). ADOS-G scores for items comprising the "communication," and "social interaction" sub-scales and the sum of both sub-scales were significantly improved after oxytocin administration. No change in ADOS-G scores related to play/imagination of restrictive/

Authors	Study Design & Participants	Oxytocin Administration and Dosage	Primary Outcomes
Guastella et al. [25]	Double-blind placebo-controlled design. 16 ASD (all male) • M_{age} = 14.88 yrs., SD_{age} = 2.42 yrs.	A single dose of oxytocin and a placebo nasal spray 1 week apart. (a) OXT nasal spray and (b) placebo containing all ingredients except active oxytocin puff per nostril contained 3 IU. Older participants (aged 16 –19, n = 5) received a dose of 24 IU (4 puffs per nostril, 3 IU per puff). Those aged 12 to 15 years n = 11 received 75% dose of the adult dose at 18 IU (3 puffs per nostril, 3 IU per puff).	Oxytocin improved performance on the REMET (particularly on "easy" items) compared to placebo.
Tachibana et al. [26]	Open label, single arm long-term design. 8 ASD (all male) • M_{age} = 11.93 yrs., SD_{age} = 1.32 yrs.	Intranasal oxytocin twice a day for approximately 7 months; dosage was increased in a stepwise fashion every 2 months (from an initial dose of 8 IU to 24 IU). Placebo was inserted between the dosing steps as a washout period. Concentration of OXT in the nasal spray was changed so that a total of 6 puffs/dose twice a day was maintained throughout the protocol.	Communication and social interaction scores on ADOS-G were significantly improved after oxytocin administration.
Anagnostou et al. [27]	Single arm, open label design. 15 ASD (11 male, 4 female) • M_{age} = 13.8 yrs., SD_{age} = 2.4 yrs.	Twice per day (morning and night) for 12 weeks; 24 IU total a day	Improvements on the following measures: ABC; SRS, BASC social skills and functional communication subscales, Let's Face It! Skills Battery, Irony and Empathy Task, Strange Stories Task, CASI, RBS-R, and C-YBOCS
Dadds et al. [28]	Double-blind, placebo controlled randomized controlled design. 38 ASD (all male). 19 in OXT group; 19 in placebo group • OXT: M_{age} = 10.74 yrs., SD_{age} = 2.38 yrs. • PLACEBO: M_{age} = 11.79 yrs., SD_{age} = 2.82 yrs.	Treatment group: intranasal spray contained: oxytocin, mannitol, glycerine, methyl parraben, propyl, parraben and purified water. Placebo contained all ingredients except the active oxytocin and mannitol. 5-day trial. Each nostril received a 12 IU dose (6 IU per puff) for a total of 24 IU/day.	No significant benefit of oxytocin versus placebo on SSRS, SRS, or an emotion recognition task.

Authors	Study Design & Participants	Oxytocin Administration and Dosage	Primary Outcomes
Guastella et al. [29]	Double-blind placebo-controlled design. 50 ASD (all male); 26 in OXT group, 24 in placebo • OXT: M_{age} = 13.85 yrs., SD_{age} = 1.54 yrs. • PLACEBO: M_{age} = 14.00 yrs., SD_{age} = 2.04 yrs.	Intranasal oxytocin or placebo, 2 times per day for 8 weeks. Older participants (aged 16 –19, n = 5 in each group) received a dose of 24 IU. Those aged 12 to 15 years received 75% of the adult dose at 18 IU.	No improvements related to oxytocin were observed on primary outcome measures (SRS or CGI-Improvement scale).
Yatawara et al. [30]	Double-blind, randomized, placebo-controlled crossover (A/B, B/A) design. 31 ASD (27 male, 4 female).15 in OXT then placebo group; 16 in placebo then OXT group • OXT first: M_{age} = 5.7 yrs., SD_{age} = 1.5 yrs. • PLACEBO first: M_{age} = 6.7 yrs., SD_{age} = 1.8 yrs.	Intranasal oxytocin or placebo twice per day for 5 weeks, followed by a 4 week wash-out period, and then received either oxytocin or placebo (whichever they did not receive in the first phase) twice per day for 5 weeks. 24 IU total per day; 12 IU in morning and 12 IU at night.	Social-communication skills (SRS) improved significantly after oxytocin versus placebo. Ratings on the CGI were significantly better after oxytocin versus placebo.
Parker et al. [22]	Double-blind, randomized, placebo-controlled design. 32 ASD (27 males, 5 females). 13 in OXT group; 14 in placebo group • OXT: M_{age} = 9.35 yrs., SD_{age} = 2.34 yrs. • PLACEBO: M_{age} = 8.13 yrs., SD_{age} = 1.87 yrs.	Treatment group: Syntocinon nasal spray; Placebo group: placebo solution consisted of all the ingredients used in the active solution except the oxytocin compound. Participants' parents then were provided with a 4-week drug supply and were responsible for their child's continued twice daily dosing (24 IU per dose, 4 IU per puff, 48 IU/day) at home.	ASD participants who received oxytocin had greater improvements on the SRS compared to ASD participants who received the placebo. Pre-treatment plasma oxytocin negatively predicted the magnitude of improvement on the SRS (i.e., participants who had lower concentrations of oxytocin pre-treatment demonstrated the largest improvements in SRS scores).
Strathearn et al. [31]	Randomized, double-blind, placebo-controlled crossover design. 16 ASD • M_{age} = 12.8 yrs., SD_{age} = 3.4 yrs. • 16 TD • M_{age} = 13.2 yrs., SD_{age} = 3.2 yrs.	One nasal solution (oxytocin or placebo) on Visit 1 and the alternate solution on Visit 2. Participants 16 years and older received 24 IU oxytocin (10 puffs alternating between nostrils 2.4 IU). Participants aged 12–15 years received 7 puffs (16.8 IU), and participants aged 8–11 years received 5 puffs (12 IU total).	After nasal oxytocin was administered to ASD participants, differences in visual preference for structured/systemized images between ASD and TD participants was eliminated.

Table 1.
Behavioral results of oxytocin administration in children with ASD.

repetitive behaviors (RRBs) were observed. No significant changes were observed for the ABC or CBCL after oxytocin administration though some scores improved at a trend level. The authors note that oxytocin administration appeared to specifically affect social communication and interaction, but did not affect RRBs or play. However, the study was open label, single arm. Therefore, caution is needed when interpreting these findings.

Anagnostou and colleagues [27] administered intranasal oxytocin to 15 male and female adolescents (ages 10-17) twice per day for 12 weeks in a single arm, open label design. Participants completed a follow-up session 12 weeks after discontinuation of oxytocin administration. Though the authors measured change on a variety of behavioral measures related to social function, social cognition, anxiety, and repetitive behaviors, the aim of the study was to measure the safety of varying dose levels of oxytocin in this population. Safety results suggested that .4 IU/kg twice per day for 12 weeks produced no serious or severe adverse events. Using the Clinical Global Improvement-Social (CGI), almost half of the sample were classified as "responders" at 12 weeks, and most responders at 12 weeks maintained improvements 12 weeks after the end of the study (e.g. 24 weeks from the beginning of the study). At 12 weeks, significant improvements were observed for the following measures: ABC [35], Social Responsiveness Scale (SRS; [37]), Behavioral Assessment System for Children (BASC; [38]) social skills and functional communication subscales, Let's Face It! Skills Battery (LFI; [39]), Irony and Empathy Task [40], Strange Stories Task [41], Child and Adolescent Symptom Inventory (CASI; [42]), Repetitive Behavior Scale-Revised (RBS-R; [43]), Child Yale-Brown Obsessive-Compulsive Scale (C-YBOCS; [44]). At 24 weeks, significant improvements were observed for the following measures: BASC functional communication T-Score, RMET [33]--difficult items, Irony and Empathy Task, and C-YBOCS. The authors note that not all children demonstrated behavioral improvements in response to oxytocin administration, and that more information is needed about individual differences in response to oxytocin. Nevertheless, a broad array of measures was, on average, shown to increase after oxytocin administration.

Dadds and colleagues [28] completed a 5-day double-blind, placebo controlled, randomized controlled trial with 38 boys with ASD (ages 7-16). This study is unique as it combined oxytocin administration with consecutive parent-child interaction training sessions over a period of 4 days. The authors did follow-up testing 3 months after the completion of the 5-day intervention. The parent-child interaction training consisted of emotion recognition training using the Mindreading (MR) program [45], and short video clips demonstrating successful client interactions (e.g. eye contact, body language, responsiveness). Outcomes included parent-child interaction tasks (free play, emotion talk, and an "I love you" task in which a parent expresses positive emotions and the child's response is recorded), and parent-questionnaire measures (Social Skills Rating Scale, or SSRS, [46]; SRS, [37]), and an emotion recognition task (UNSW Facial Emotion Task, [28]). Analysis of the parent-child interaction tasks, parent rating scales, and emotion recognition tasks indicated behavioral improvements over time in both the placebo and oxytocin groups, but no significant benefit of oxytocin versus placebo. We note that although this study combined oxytocin and behavioral intervention, the intervention was not one previously validated for improving core symptoms of ASD, and the study timeline was short (5 days).

Guastella and colleagues [29] completed a double-blind placebo-controlled trial with 50 male participants with ASD (ages 12-18). Participants received either placebo or oxytocin nasal spray twice a day for 8 weeks. Participants were assessed again 3 months after completion of the study. Primary outcome measures were the SRS [37] and clinician ratings on the Clinical Global Impressions--Improvement scale

(CGI-Improvement). Secondary outcome measures included the Developmental Behaviour Checklist, or DBC [47] and Repetitive Behavior Scale-Revised, or RBS [43], RMET [33], the Diagnostic analysis of nonverbal accuracy, or DANVA [48], and Biological Motion [49]. No improvements related to oxytocin were observed on the primary or secondary outcome measures.

Yatawara and colleagues [30] completed a double-blind, randomized, placebo-controlled crossover (A/B, B/A) design trial in 31 children with ASD (ages 3-8). Children received intranasal oxytocin or placebo twice per day for 5 weeks, completed a 4-week wash-out period, and then received either oxytocin or placebo (whichever they did not receive in the first phase) twice per day for 5 weeks. Primary outcome measures were scores on the SRS [37], and scores on the RBS-R [43]. Secondary outcome measures were changes in ADOS scores, scores on the DBC [50], clinician-rated clinical global impressions-improvement scale [51], and the Caregiver Strain Questionnaire [52]. Results indicated that parent-rated social-communication skills (SRS) improved significantly after oxytocin versus placebo. Ratings on the CGI were significantly better after oxytocin versus placebo. To our knowledge, this study includes the youngest sample of children with ASD to receive oxytocin versus placebo in a randomized, double-blind trial. This work provides behavioral evidence of symptom reduction in ASD in response to prolonged oxytocin administration.

Parker and colleagues [22] completed a double-blind, randomized, placebo-controlled trial with 32 children with ASD (ages 6-12). Children received either intranasal oxytocin or placebo twice per day for 4 weeks. The primary outcome measure was scores on the SRS [37]. Secondary outcome measures included scores on the RBS-R [43] and Spence Children's Anxiety Scale [53]. Additionally, authors measured plasma oxytocin concentrations both before and after participation in the trial, as well as expression of genes related to oxytocin receptors (Oxytocin Receptor Gene, OXTR, and Vasopressin Receptor 1a; V1AR). Results suggested that children who received oxytocin demonstrated greater improvements on the SRS compared to those receiving placebo. Additionally, pre-treatment plasma oxytocin negatively predicted the magnitude of improvement on the SRS. That is, individuals who had the lowest concentrations of oxytocin pre-treatment demonstrated the largest improvements. The authors hypothesized conflicting findings of previous oxytocin trials may be attributable to variability in pre-treatment concentrations of oxytocin. That is, previous trials did not measure pre-treatment oxytocin concentrations which may have reduced their ability to accurately measure improvement. When the authors did not include pre-treatment oxytocin, concentration findings were non-significant. In fact, inclusion of these pre-treatment "biomarkers" improved the statistical models by 43%, which underscores the importance of measuring individual variability in pre-post measurement designs.

Strathearn and colleagues [31] completed a double-blind, placebo-controlled crossover study with 16 children with ASD and 16 neurotypical children (ages 8-19). Participants completed an eye tracking paradigm on two occasions: once after receiving oxytocin and the other after receiving a placebo nasal spray. The authors measured participants' eye gaze while viewing images that varied on how organized or structured they were. The authors' primary focus was whether or not oxytocin affected eye gaze patterns when viewing stimuli that varied on levels of systemization. Results demonstrated that after oxytocin administration, children and adolescents with ASD displayed a decreased preference for highly systemized stimuli, whereas neurotypical children and adolescents displayed increased preference for systemized images. Overall, when participants received placebo, children and adolescents with ASD displayed more of a preference for systemized stimuli compared to their neurotypical peers. After both groups received oxytocin this difference was no longer significant (e.g. participants with ASD looked more similar to their neurotypical peers, and neurotypical children and teens looked more similar to their peers with ASD). The authors concluded that oxytocin administration may have differential effects on individuals with and without ASD, but that oxytocin appears to decrease preference for highly organized (e.g. systemized) stimuli in ASD.

Overall, studies of the behavioral effects of oxytocin in children in ASD are mixed, with some investigations observing significant behavioral changes [22, 25–27, 30, 31], whereas others find no evidence for change as a function of oxytocin versus placebo administration [28, 29]. A likely explanation for these disparate findings is outlined by Parker and colleagues [22]. The authors noted that measuring participant's plasma oxytocin levels provided a critical "biomarker" for predicting a given individual's response to oxytocin administration. Most studies do not measure oxytocin concentration prior to administration and therefore may miss individual differences which significantly impact outcomes. Parker and colleagues [22] noted that without the addition of pre-administration plasma oxytocin concentration into their predictive models, their results would have indicated no difference between oxytocin and placebo. When pre-administration oxytocin levels were included, their models were improved by 43%. This underscores why it is critical to consider biological differences in individuals *prior* to administration of oxytocin in order to more accurately understand variability within samples of children with ASD. When such individual differences are considered, behavioral effects of oxytocin may be more detectable, and/or may help us understand which children are most likely to benefit from oxytocin.

4.2 Neuroscience findings

To our knowledge, only 3 studies have investigated the effects of oxytocin on brain activity in children with ASD [54–56]; see [57] for a review. See **Table 2**.

Gordon and colleagues [54] used functional magnetic resonance imaging (fMRI) to measure brain activity after oxytocin versus placebo in 17 children and adolescents with ASD (ages 8-16.5) using a randomized, double-blind, crossover design. Forty-five minutes after administration of either oxytocin or placebo, participants completed an fMRI emotion recognition task based on the RMET [33]. In a control fMRI condition, participants were asked to label the category of automobile presented in pictures. Findings suggested enhanced brain activity after oxytocin administration in brain areas hypothesized to be critical to reward (dorsal and ventral striatum), social attention and cognition (posterior cingulate, inferior parietal lobule, posterior superior temporal sulcus), and reasoning about mental states (medial prefrontal cortex). In addition, several brain regions were less active during nonsocial judgements after oxytocin administration. Interestingly, the effect of oxytocin on brain activity in response to social judgements differed as a function of symptom severity. Children with ASD with less severe symptoms (measured with the SRS) exhibited more 'typical' brain activity after oxytocin administration compared to children with ASD with more severe symptoms. Taken together, the authors hypothesized that oxytocin may increase the reward value and/or salience of social stimuli for children with ASD while simultaneously decreasing the salience of nonsocial information.

Gordon and colleagues [55] employed a randomized, double-blind, placebo-controlled crossover design with 20 children with ASD (ages 8-16.5). Participants completed an fMRI scan twice: once receiving oxytocin and the other after receiving placebo nasal spray. The authors measured participants' brain activity in response to two social perception tasks: a biological motion task and an affective voices task. The authors' primary aim was to measure whether oxytocin increased brain activity in areas related to the reward system and the connections between reward and social brain regions

Authors	Participants and Oxytocin Administration	Design and Stimuli/ Paradigm	Major Findings
Gordon et al. [54]	21 ASD (3 females; 18 males) • M_{age} = 13.2 yrs., SD_{age} = 2.7 yrs. Intranasally. Older participants (16 – 19 yrs.) received a dose of 24 IU (4 puffs per nostril); 15 yr olds received 18 IU (3 puffs per nostril); Younger participants (7 - 11 yrs.) received 12 IUs, (1 puff per nostril); or placebo. Testing was repeated on consecutive study visits. Order was randomized.	Randomized, double-blind, cross-over design. fMRI. Reading the Mind in the Eyes Test (RMET). Participants were instructed to label the mental state of each facial picture, or label the category of automobile images.	Social condition: Enhanced activity in the dorsal and ventral striatum, premotor cortex, posterior cingulate, inferior parietal lobule, and posterior STS in response to oxytocin compared to placebo.
Gordon et al. [55]	20 ASD (3 females) • M_{age} = 13.2 yrs., SD_{age} = 2.8 yrs. Intranasally. Older participants (16 – 19 yrs.) received a dose of 24 IU (4 puffs per nostril); 15 yr olds received 18 IU (3 puffs per nostril). Younger participants (7 - 11 yrs.) received 12 IUs, (1 puff per nostril); or placebo. Testing was repeated on consecutive study visits. Placebo or oxytocin was randomized at the first visit and participants received the opposite nasal spray at the second visit.	Randomized, double blind, placebo-controlled crossover design. fMRI. Participants passively viewed a biological motion paradigm (human motion and scrambled motion) and listened to a vocal affect perception paradigm (angry voices and happy voices).	Biological motion condition: enhanced response in the right posterior superior temporal sulcus (pSTS) after oxytocin compared to placebo administration. Negative vocal affect condition: Enhanced activation in right brainstem and right amygdala after oxytocin versus placebo administration.
Greene et al. [56]	28 ASD (2 females, 26 males) • M_{age} = 13.4 yrs., SD_{age} = 2.4 yrs. Intranasally. 3 puffs per nostril (Syntocinon), each puff contained 4 IU of oxytocin, for a total of 24 IU, or placebo containing the same inactive ingredients. Nostrils were alternated between puffs over the course of several minutes. Two scan sessions were scheduled at least 72 hours apart from one another. Order of oxytocin and placebo were counter-balanced.	Placebo-controlled double-blind design. fMRI. Participants completed an incentive delay task with nonsocial (money) or social rewards (smiling face).	Anticipation of nonsocial reward: Increased activity in right nucleus accumbens (NAcc), right frontal pole, left ACC, left superior frontal cortex, bilateral orbital frontal cortex (OFC) after oxytocin versus placebo administration. Increased functional connectivity during nonsocial reward anticipation (between the right NAcc and the right FP) after oxytocin versus placebo. Nonsocial reward outcome: Decreased frontostriatal functional connectivity between left ACC, bilateral postcentral gyrus, left inferior front gyrus, left precentral gyrus, and left medial frontal gyrus after oxytocin vs placebo administration.

Table 2.
Neuroscience results after oxytocin administration in children with ASD.

(e.g. mesocorticolimbic pathways and communication between this pathway and socially-relevant brain regions) compared to placebo. Results were consistent with the author's hypotheses: oxytocin enhanced neural responses to biological versus random motion in the posterior superior temporal sulcus (pSTS), and in the amygdala and hippocampus in response to angry versus happy voices. Across both fMRI tasks, oxytocin increased neural connectivity both within reward regions and between the reward pathway and regions associated with social perception. The authors concluded that oxytocin administration appeared to enhance salience/reward of social stimuli (as measured in the biological motion task), but also increased the salience of negative social stimuli (as measured by the affective voices task).

Greene and colleagues [56] conducted a placebo-controlled, double-blind study with 28 children and adolescents with ASD (ages 10-17). Participants completed an fMRI incentive delay task on two occasions: once after receiving oxytocin, and once after receiving a placebo nasal spray. The fMRI task involved both social and non-social reward conditions so the authors could compare the effects of oxytocin versus placebo on brain activity related to both social and nonsocial rewards. Results demonstrated that compared to placebo, oxytocin increased brain activity in the caudate nucleus, left anterior cingulate cortex, frontal pole, insular cortex, and orbito-frontal cortex in the nonsocial reward versus social reward condition. Additionally, the authors found a positive relationship between symptom severity (measured using the SRS; [37]) and activation in the frontal pole and anterior cingulate during nonsocial reward anticipation, and between symptom severity and activation in the precentral gyrus and left caudate during nonsocial reward processing. Interestingly, these findings do not support the hypothesis that oxytocin selectively enhances reward-related brain activity to social stimuli, but rather may be associated with increased reward anticipation and processing for nonsocial stimuli. The authors hypothesize that reward-related effects of oxytocin may be sensitive to task-specific features, and noted that their findings strengthen the body of evidence that oxytocin acts on the brain's reward system.

Taken together, these findings provide further evidence that intranasal oxytocin administration appears to act on the neural reward system. However, evidence is mixed regarding whether oxytocin specifically acts on the social reward system [54, 55] or the reward system more broadly [56]. It is likely that differences in neuroscience tasks, as well as differences in regions of interest, and participant sample characteristics may explain disparate findings. Importantly for our theoretical framework, intranasal oxytocin administration appears to impact the reward system in children with ASD. This provides an empirical basis for our hypothesis that combining a pharmacological agent with behavioral interventions that act on similar brain regions/networks may improve outcomes related to social initiation and communication.

5. Behavioral Interventions in ASD

Given the heterogeneous behavioral manifestations of ASD, it is not surprising that multiple behavioral interventions have been developed to improve social communication and decrease challenging behaviors [58–60]. Multiple systematic reviews have been published on the success of behavioral interventions for children with ASD (e.g. [61–64]), and an extensive review is beyond the scope of the current chapter. Of primary relevance to the current chapter are behavioral interventions designed to increase the salience, relevance, and reward value of social interactions in order to improve social-communicative symptoms.

This section will briefly review two of these behavioral interventions, specifically the Early Start Denver Model (ESDM) and Pivotal Response Training (PRT) as both of these interventions are based on principles of Applied Behavioral Analysis (ABA) but emphasize naturalistic teaching strategies to promote generalization. Note, however, that there are other naturalistic interventions grounded in ABA principles (e.g. Incidental Teaching [65]; Reciprocal Imitation Training, or RIT [66, 67]; Parent-training programs, such as Project ImPACT [68]; Joint attention Interventions, such as JASPER [69, 70], and others).

5.1 Early start denver model (ESDM)

ESDM is an empirically validated, manualized intensive early intervention program designed for children between the ages of 1-4 [60, 71]. ESDM uses teaching strategies including: interpersonal exchange and positive affect, engagement with real-world activities and materials, adult responsivity and sensitivity, and focus on both verbal and nonverbal communication. These strategies are grounded in ABA principles including operant conditioning, shaping, and chaining. Importantly, ESDM is not conceptualized as a behavioral intervention that must occur in a table-top or structured situation, nor is it a "one size fits all" approach. Each child's program is individualized, and parent's roles are emphasized. Parents are taught ESDM strategies and encouraged to utilize them during daily activities (e.g. feeding, bath time, play). In a 2010 randomized controlled trial, Dawson and colleagues compared the efficacy of ESDM versus treatment as usual (TAU) over a 2-year period [60]. Results found significant improvements in cognitive abilities in the ESDM group compared to TAU. These group differences appeared driven by improvements in both expressive and receptive language in the ESDM group. Additionally, significant group differences were observed in adaptive behaviors. Whereas children in the ESDM group remained steady in their adaptive behaviors across time, children in the TAU group exhibited lower scores across time when compared to their neurotypical peers. This difference appeared driven by increasing gaps between the TAU group and their neurotypical peers in a variety of adaptive skills, whereas children in the ESDM group displayed improvement in their communication abilities. A recent meta-analysis corroborates the efficacy of ESDM in improving cognition and language for children with ASD [72].

5.2 Pivotal response training (PRT)

Pivotal response training (PRT), sometimes referred to as Pivotal Response Teaching or Pivotal Response Therapy, is a naturalistic behavior intervention based on principles of ABA. The underlying assumption of PRT is that children's challenges can be improved with behavioral and environmental manipulations including reinforcement, contingencies, consequences, and extinction [73]. The term "pivotal" is important as it refers to pivotal behaviors that, when targeted, can lead to improvements in other areas of behavior not specifically targeted. The behaviors/function areas most commonly targeted in PRT are: motivation, initiation, responding to multiple cues, and self-management [74, 75]. To increase motivation, teaching strategies include: following the child's lead, offering choices, providing clear opportunities for response, varying tasks, including both maintenance and acquisition tasks, contingent and natural reinforcement, and reinforcing all attempts at target skills [73, 74]. Similar to ESDM, PRT emphasizes the importance of implementing the intervention in the child's natural environment and the involvement of parents and other caregivers in the intervention [73]. Results of a systematic review indicate that PRT is largely effective at increasing self-initiation and improving language, communication, and play skills in children with ASD [76]. A 2016 meta-analysis concluded that PRT is effective at teaching behaviors to children with ASD [77].

6. Neuroscience findings after behavioral intervention in ASD

Despite a wealth of research examining the behavioral utility of empirically-based interventions for children with ASD, there is a relative paucity of literature utilizing neuroscience as an outcome measure or predictor of behavioral intervention response (see [78] for a review). To our knowledge, seven studies have been published using neuroscience as either an outcome measure or predictor of response for an empirically supported behavioral intervention designed to help with core symptoms of ASD. See **Table 3**.

The first published paper using neuroscience as an outcome measure was Dawson and colleagues in 2012 [79]. 29 children with ASD (ages 48-77 months) participated in the study and were randomly assigned to either receive two years of ESDM intervention or two years of treatment as usual, TAU. Compared to toddlers in the community intervention, those who received ESDM demonstrated faster neural signatures of attention (the Nc ERP component) when viewing faces versus objects. Interestingly, when brain activity patterns of the two groups of toddlers with ASD were compared to brain activity of neurotypical (TD) toddlers, the ESDM and TD groups exhibited increased cortical activation when viewing faces versus objects, whereas toddlers in the TAU group evidenced more cortical activation when viewing objects vs. faces. The authors concluded that participation in ESDM appeared to lead to "normalization" of attention to faces. However, the authors did not include measures of brain activity prior to intervention, so they were unable to directly infer whether participation in ESDM significantly changed brain activity from pre to post intervention.

Voos and colleagues [80] used fMRI to measure brain activity in two five-year-olds with ASD before and after four months of PRT. The fMRI paradigm involved watching point-light displays that were either attached to an adult who performed actions (e.g. biological motion) or scrambled light displays created with random selections of light points (scrambled motion). When measuring brain activity from brain areas implicated in ASD from previous research [81], the authors found that one participant had increased brain activity after intervention in the left fusiform gyrus and left dorsal prefrontal cortex, and the other participant had greater activation in the left ventrolateral prefrontal cortex, right posterior superior temporal sulcus, and fusiform gyrus. All of these brain regions have been previously implicated as relevant to processing social stimuli and biological motion. Despite the small sample size, the results suggest that PRT can increase brain activity in important regions associated with social stimuli.

Ventola and colleagues [82] also measured brain activity before and after participation in PRT. 10 children with ASD (aged 4-7) completed an fMRI biological motion task both before and after 16 weeks of PRT. 5 neurotypical children were tested twice (once at "baseline" and once 16 weeks later) but they did not receive PRT. Based on activity in the parietal temporal sulcus (pSTS) at baseline compared to neurotypical participants, children with ASD were separated into two groups: hypo- and hyper-active. Children with hypo-activation were hypothesized to have decreased social motivation (evidenced by hypoactivity in the pSTS compared to neurotypical children), and children with hyper-activation were hypothesized to be hypersensitive to stimuli (evidenced by hyperactivity in the pSTS compared to neurotypical children). After PRT, children in the hypo-active

Authors	Participants	Intervention, Neuroscience Methodology, & Task	Neuroscientific Findings
Dawson et al. [79]	15 ASD in ESDM group • M_{age} = 54.1 mo., SD_{age} = 4.9 mo. 14 ASD in the TAU group • M_{age} = 54.1 mo., SD_{age} = 7.8 mo. 17 TD participants • M_{age} = 55.7 mo., SD_{age} = 4.5 mo.	ESDM; 2 for years; 20 hours/ week ERP Participants viewed images of faces and toys.	Faster Nc and increased cortical activation to faces vs. objects in the EDSM group. Faster Nc and increased cortical activation to objects vs. faces in the TAU group.
Voos et al. [80]	2 ASD (1 male, 1 female), each 5 years old	PRT; 16 weeks; 8– 10 hours/ week fMRI Participants viewed biological motion clips and scrambled motion clips.	During biological motion: Participant 1 (female): Increased activity in the fusiform gyrus (FG) and dorsolateral prefrontal cortex (dlPFC). Participant 2 (male): Increased activity in the posterior superior temporal sulcus (pSTS), ventrolateral prefrontal cortex (vlPFC), and FG.
Ventola et al. [82]	10 ASD (8 male, 2 female) Hypoactive group (3 male, 2 female): • M_{age} = 5.3 yrs., SD_{age} = .27 yrs. Hyperactive group (5 male): • M_{age} = 5.66 yrs., SD_{age} = 1.02 yrs.	PRT; 16 weeks; 7 hours/week fMRI Participants viewed biological motion clips and scrambled motion clips.	During biological motion: Initially hypoactive group: increased activation in the ventral striatum (VS) and right posterior superior temporal sulcus (pSTS) Initially hyperactive group: decreased activation in right pSTS, amygdala, thalamus, and hippocampus.
Van Hecke et al. [83]	28 ASD in the immediate treatment group (22 male, 6 female) • M_{age} = 14.1 yrs., SD_{age} = 1.3 yrs. 29 ASD in the waitlist control (WLC) group (23 male, 6 female) • M_{age} = 13.3 yrs., SD_{age} = 1.7 yrs. 30 TD (28 male, 2 female) • M_{age} = 13.3 yrs., SD_{age} = 1.3 yrs.	PEERS; 14 weeks; 1.5 hours/week EEG Continuous resting EEG	Immediate treatment: Increased left-dominant gamma asymmetry during resting state EEG after intervention vs. pre-intervention (more similar to TD). WLC: no change.
Venkataraman et al. [88]	19 ASD (13 males, 6 females) • M_{age} = 5.87 yrs., SD_{age} = 1.09 yrs.	PRT; 16 weeks; 7 hours/week fMRI Participants viewed biological motion clips and scrambled motion clips.	During biological motion, reduction in connectivity between the posterior cingulate cortex (PCC) and orbital frontal cortex and an increase in connectivity between the PCC and regions of ventral occipital temporal extrastriate cortex.

Authors	Participants	Intervention, Neuroscience Methodology, & Task	Neuroscientific Findings
Yang et al. [89]	20 ASD (13 male, 7 female) • M_{age} = 5.90 yrs., SD_{age} = 1.07 yrs.	PRT; 16 weeks; 7 hours/week fMRI Participants viewed biological motion clips and scrambled motion clips.	Pre-intervention brain activity in the following areas while viewing biological motion predicted behavioral improvements on the SRS from pre- to post-intervention. (1) social perception (fusiform gyrus, inferior temporal gyrus, middle temporal gyrus), (2) social attention (inferior parietal gyrus, superior parietal lobule), (3) emotion regulation and reward (orbitofrontal cortex, ventrolateral prefrontal cortex, anterior insula), and (4) social reward (putamen, pallidum, amygdala, hippocampus, ventral striatum)
Baker et al., [90]	7 ASD (6 male, 1 female) • M_{age} = 13.88 yrs., SD_{age} = 2.21 yrs. 7 TD (6 male, 1 female) • M_{age} = 13.46 yrs., SD_{age} = 2.29 yrs.	PEERS; 16 weeks; 1.5 hours/week ERP Participants completed a reward task with feedback that was social (face) or nonsocial (arrow) with correct or incorrect feedback (face: smile vs frown; arrow: upward vs downward).	Increased neural sensitivity to both social and nonsocial rewards (RewP amplitude) after versus before intervention.

Table 3.
Neuroscience outcome measures of behavioral interventions in children with ASD.

group had increased brain activity in the pSTS and ventral striatum when viewing biological motion, and decreased ventral striatum activity in response to scrambled motion. Children in the hyperactive group evidenced decreased brain activity in the pSTS, amygdala, thalamus, and hippocampus when viewing biological motion. The authors' hypothesized that participation in PRT differentially affected brain activity of children depending on their baseline characteristics (e.g. children who displayed too little brain activity in response to social stimuli evidenced increased brain activity after intervention, whereas children who displayed too much brain activity in response to social stimuli evidenced decreased activity after intervention).

Van Hecke and colleagues [83] used electrophysiology (EEG) to measure brain activity before and after participation in a randomized control trial of the Program for the Education and Enrichment of Relational Skills (PEERS; [84, 85]) versus a waitlist control (WLC) condition. PEERS is an empirically validated, manualized program which focuses on making and keeping friends for adolescents with ASD [86].

35 adolescents (13-14 years old) with ASD were randomly assigned to receive PEERS, 31 were randomly assigned to WLC, and 30 neurotypical (TD) adolescents were assessed prior to the intervention for comparison purposes. The authors measured brain activity patterns during "resting state" during which adolescents were instructed to focus on a fixation point for three minutes. Of particular interest was patterns of brain activity in the right versus left hemispheres as previous research suggests that individuals who have left-hemisphere dominance have higher approach motivation and positive affect compared to those with right-hemisphere dominance who are often characterized as withdrawn [87]. Prior to intervention, the two groups of teens with ASD evidenced less left-dominant asymmetry compared to the TD group. When comparing post-intervention brain activity of teens who received PEERS to brain activity in the TD group, differences in left-hemispheric dominance were no longer observed. Differences between the WLC group and the TD group were still observed after the 14-week intervention period (during which the WLC group did not receive intervention). These findings suggest that participation in PEERS (compared to a waitlist condition) significantly changed patterns of brain activity to be increasingly left-hemisphere dominant, which is more similar to patterns observed in neurotypical teens.

Venkataraman and colleagues [88] used a Bayesian probabilistic model to characterize fMRI activity in 19 children with ASD (mean age 5.87 years) before and after 16 weeks of PRT. Similar to Ventola et al. [82], the fMRI paradigm involved watching two types of light displays: biological motion and scrambled motion. The probabilistic model allowed the authors to measure PRT-induced changes in neural connectivity between neural regions of interest. Results indicated both reduced connectivity between the posterior cingulate cortex (PCC) and orbitofrontal cortex and increased connectivity between the PCC and areas of the ventral occipital temporal extrastriate cortex. These results are interesting given that the PCC is known for its role in social cognitive processes, the orbitofrontal cortex has been implicated in reward processes, and the ventral occipital and temporal cortices play a role in processing socially meaningful stimuli (including biological motion). These findings suggest that PRT causes a shift, in which connectivity between the PCC and orbitofrontal cortex is decreased while PCC and the ventral occipital-temporal cortex connection is strengthened.

Yang and colleagues [89] utilized fMRI as a pre-intervention predictor of intervention response in 20 children with ASD (mean age 5.90 years). The authors measured brain activity during a biological motion paradigm prior to 16 weeks of PRT. Results demonstrated that pre-intervention brain activity in areas implicated in: (1) social perception (fusiform gyrus, inferior temporal gyrus, middle temporal gyrus), (2) social attention (inferior parietal gyrus, superior parietal lobule), (3) emotion regulation and reward (orbitofrontal cortex, ventrolateral prefrontal cortex, anterior insula), and (4) social reward (putamen, pallidum, amygdala, hippocampus, ventral striatum) while viewing biological motion predicted behavioral improvements on the SRS from pre- to post-intervention. For all 4 regions, greater levels of pre-intervention brain activity were associated with increased behavioral improvements from pre- to post- intervention. Results from this study suggest that neuroscience methods may be able to predict which children are most likely to benefit from a specific intervention, as well as underscoring the importance of brain regions associated with social perception, emotion regulation, and reward for understanding how interventions may affect brain circuitry in ASD.

Baker and colleagues [90] used event-related potentials (ERP) to measure brain response to reward in ASD adolescents before and after participation in the PEERS program compared to a typically developing sample. Response to social and nonsocial rewards were measured using the reward-related positive component (RewP) in seven adolescents with ASD and seven TD adolescents, aged 10 to 17 years. Prior to intervention, patterns of reward-related brain activity (RewP mean amplitude) did not differ between groups. However, after intervention the ASD group demonstrated an enhanced sensitivity to rewards, regardless of social or nonsocial condition, compared to the TD group. Additionally, ASD participants with less robust responses to social rewards prior to the start of the PEERS intervention demonstrated the most gains in social behaviors (as measured via SRS-2 [91]; Social Skills Improvement System, [92]. Findings from this study suggest an enhancement of the neural response to rewards after teens with ASD receive training in social skills and additionally that teens with attenuated responses to social rewards may gain the most benefit from intervention.

Taken together, these seven studies provide evidence for two critical concepts: (1) *Behavioral Intervention* can significantly change patterns and/or magnitude of brain activity in response to social stimuli for children with ASD, and (2) *Neuroscience* may be able to predict individual levels of behavioral intervention response and could eventually be used to advance "precision medicine" (e.g. to predict who is most likely to benefit from a specific intervention). The first concept is central to our theoretical framework, as it suggests that participation in empirically based interventions changes brain activity in children with ASD--particularly in response to social stimuli and in brain areas/patterns of activity related to social perception and reward. Neural changes in the reward system and other areas of the "social brain" after interventions provides an empirical basis for our hypothesis that the addition of pharmacological compounds that enhance brain activity/responses in those same regions might lead to increased benefits for children with ASD.

7. Current research combining oxytocin and behavioral interventions in ASD

Although there are no published studies (to our knowledge) that have conducted double-blind, placebo-controlled trials combining oxytocin administration with an empirically validated behavioral intervention in ASD, two trials are currently underway and recorded on ClinicalTrials.Gov (identifiers NCT02918864 and NCT03370510). We also note that a large-scale multi-site trial of the behavioral effects of oxytocin versus placebo is underway by the Study of Oxytocin in Autism to Improve Reciprocal Social Behaviors (SOARS-B; clinical trial identifier NCT01944046). One paper describing the rationale and methods for the trial has been published [93].

8. Does timing matter?

As noted above, we hypothesize that empirically based behavioral interventions designed to increase social-communication skills such as social initiation/motivation are more likely to be enhanced by oxytocin administration than interventions focused on other aspects of ASD (e.g. disruptive behaviors, anxiety). Such interventions are typically aimed towards young children (i.e. ESDM was developed for children ages 1-4) due to the targeted skills. We hypothesize that age is likely to play an important role in the efficacy of combining oxytocin with behavioral interventions such that younger children are more likely to benefit due to: (a) Early interventions in ASD often focus on improving social motivation and initiation, whereas interventions for older children are less likely to have such an emphasis. As oxytocin has been shown to affect the reward system, behavioral interventions designed to increase the reward value of social stimuli are likely to be the best candidates for this framework. (b) Increased neural plasticity in younger ages and the negative neuro-developmental sequelae described in the social motivation hypothesis. That is, young children have been hypothesized to benefit more from early intervention for ASD compared to older children due to neural plasticity, and the social motivation hypothesis posits that decreased reward value of social stimuli early in life leads to a negative cascade of developmental consequences [5, 94]. It therefore seems likely that younger children are best positioned to benefit from combining behavioral intervention with oxytocin because early interventions may disrupt this negative developmental cascade and help children move back towards a typical trajectory. (c) Accumulating evidence that interventions for ASD are likely to be more effective if started earlier in life [94–96]. It is unclear, however, exactly how age will affect our theoretical model. Future research should pay close attention to how and if age is a predictor when measuring outcomes of combining oxytocin and behavioral intervention in ASD.

9. Conclusions

Taken together, considering extant research findings from behavioral and neural effects of oxytocin administration along with those on brain activity in response to behavioral interventions in children with ASD suggests that both oxytocin and behavioral interventions lead to measurable changes in regions of the “social brain” and reward network. These findings, combined with those suggesting that oxytocin administration may improve social-communication in children with ASD, provide the empirical basis of our hypothesis [57] that combining oxytocin administration with behavioral interventions may improve outcomes related to social-communication. We hypothesize that the administration of oxytocin prior to each session of an intervention may “prime” the neural reward system to be maximally responsive to the behavioral skills taught during the intervention session. Due to the central role of the reward system in our theoretical model we hypothesize that this combined approach may be most effective for social-communicative skills requiring social motivation (e.g. social initiation/approach) and be maximally beneficial for young children. See **Figure 1** for hypothesized neural mechanisms underlying the efficacy of combining interventions with oxytocin to improve outcomes.

It is important to note, however, that this approach is unlikely to be equally effective in all children with ASD. As with all interventions, there does not appear to be any “one size fits all” approach to help children with ASD. It will be critical to measure and characterize individual differences that may explain variability in treatment efficacy from *biological* (e.g. levels of oxytocin concentration in plasma/saliva before and after oxytocin administration, genetic expression of candidate genes relevant for oxytocin; OXTR, VAP1, brain activity in response to social stimuli prior to oxytocin administration, age), *behavioral* (e.g. social communicative symptom profile prior to oxytocin administration), and *psychological* (e.g. co-occurring diagnoses such as ADHD, anxiety, etc.) standpoints. Such individual differences will likely be central to our understanding of how, why, and for whom this combined approach will be maximally effective.

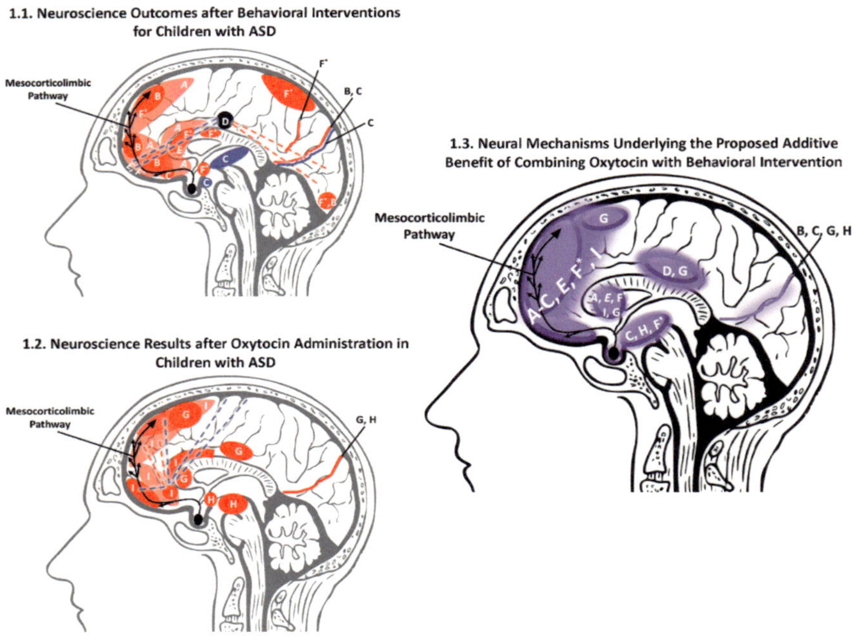

Figure 1
(1.1) Neuroscience Outcomes after Behavioral Intervention for Children with ASD. This figure depicts results from studies which measured brain activity before and after behavioral intervention. The brain areas highlighted in red indicate increased brain activity after behavioral intervention, whereas regions shown in blue indicate decreased brain activity after behavioral intervention. Results related to neural connectivity are shown with a dotted line. A. Dawson et al. [79], proposed neural generators of the Nc component (Reynolds & Richards, 2005) are highlighted (medial frontal gyrus, inferior frontal gyrus, anterior cingulate cortex); B. Voos et al. [80] (fusiform gyrus, dorsolateral prefrontal cortex, posterior superior temporal sulcus (pSTS), ventrolateral prefrontal cortex (vlPFC)); C. Ventola et al. [82], ventral striatum (VS), pSTS, amygdala, thalamus, and hippocampus; D. Venkataraman et al. [88], reduction in connectivity between the posterior cingulate cortex (PCC) and orbital frontal cortex (OFC) and an increase in connectivity between the PCC and regions of ventral occipital temporal extrastriate cortex; E. Baker et al. [90], proposed neural generators of the RewP component (Carlson et al., 2011 & Proudfit, 2015) are highlighted (ventral striatum, dorsal striatum, OFC, medial frontal cortex); F. Yang et al. [89], activity in the following pre-intervention brain areas were used to predict behavioral improvements: fusiform gyrus, inferior temporal gyrus, middle temporal gyrus, inferior parietal gyrus, superior parietal lobule, OFC, ventrolateral prefrontal cortex, anterior insula, putamen, pallidum, amygdala, hippocampus, ventral striatum. *This study used neuroscience measures prior to intervention as a predictor of intervention success, whereas the other studies used neuroscience measures pre- and post-intervention. (1.2) Neuroscience Results after Oxytocin Administration in Children with ASD. This figure depicts results from studies that have measured brain activity after oxytocin administration. Results related to neural connectivity are shown with a dotted line (red dotted line indicates increased connectivity, blue dotted line indicates decreased connectivity). G. Gordon et al., [55] (dorsal and ventral striatum, premotor cortex, posterior cingulate, pSTS); H. Gordon et al. [56] (pSTS, right amygdala, right brain stem); I. Greene et al., [56] (right nucleus accumbens (NAcc), right frontal pole (FP), left anterior cingulate cortex (ACC), left superior frontal cortex, bilateral OFC, functional connectivity during nonsocial reward anticipation (between the right NAcc and the right FP); frontostriatal functional connectivity between left ACC, bilateral postcentral gyrus, left inferior front gyrus, left precentral gyrus, and left medial frontal gyrus). (1.3) Neural Mechanisms Underlying the Proposed Additive Benefit of Combining Oxytocin with Behavioral Intervention. This figure depicts the proposed additive benefits of combining oxytocin administration with behavioral interventions for children with ASD. Brain regions that have been implicated in both behavioral intervention and oxytocin administration are labeled. We propose that oxytocin administration will "prime" neural structures related to reward and/or social information processing, which will make behavioral intervention sessions more effective.*

Author details

Katherine Kuhl Meltzoff Stavropoulos* and Elizabeth Baker
University of California, Riverside, Riverside, California, USA

*Address all correspondence to: katherine.stavropoulos@ucr.edu

References

[1] Maenner M J 2020 Prevalence of autism spectrum disorder among children aged 8 years — autism and developmental disabilities monitoring network, 11 sites, United States, 2016 *MMWR Surveill Summ* **69**

[2] American Psychiatric Association 2013 *Diagnostic and statistical manual of mental disorders* (Washington, DC: American Psychiatric Publishing)

[3] Dawson G, Webb S J and McPartland J 2005 Understanding the nature of face processing impairment in autism: insights from behavioral and electrophysiological studies *Dev Neuropsychol* **27** 403-24

[4] Chevallier C, Kohls G, Troiani V, Brodkin E S and Schultz R T 2012 The social motivation theory of autism *Trends Cogn Sci* **16** 231-9

[5] Dawson G 2008 Early behavioral intervention, brain plasticity, and the prevention of autism spectrum disorder *Dev Psychopathol* **20** 775-803

[6] Stavropoulos K K M and Carver L J 2013 Research Review: Social motivation and oxytocin in autism – implications for joint attention development and intervention *Journal of Child Psychology and Psychiatry* **54** 603-18

[7] Gainer H, Altstein M and Whitnall M H 1987 The cell biology and development of vasopressinergic and oxytocinergic neurons *Prog. Brain Res.* **72** 153-61

[8] Magon N and Kalra S 2011 The orgasmic history of oxytocin: Love, lust, and labor *Indian J Endocrinol Metab* **15** S156-61

[9] Carter C S and Porges S W 2013 The biochemistry of love: An oxytocin hypothesis *EMBO reports* **14** 12-6

[10] Modi M E and Young L J 2012 The oxytocin system in drug discovery for autism: Animal models and novel therapeutic strategies *Horm Behav* **61** 340-50

[11] Domes G, Heinrichs M, Michel A, Berger C and Herpertz S C 2007 Oxytocin improves "mind-reading" in humans *Biological Psychiatry* **61** 731-3

[12] Hurlemann R, Patin A, Onur O A, Cohen M X, Baumgartner T, Metzler S, Dziobek I, Gallinat J, Wagner M, Maier W and Kendrick K M 2010 Oxytocin enhances amygdala-dependent, socially reinforced learning and emotional empathy in humans *J. Neurosci.* **30** 4999-5007

[13] Kosfeld M, Heinrichs M, Zak P J, Fischbacher U and Fehr E 2005 Oxytocin increases trust in humans *Nature* **435** 673-6

[14] Gordon I, Martin C, Feldman R and Leckman J F 2011 Oxytocin and social motivation *Dev Cogn Neurosci* **1** 471-93

[15] Baskerville T A and Douglas A J 2010 Dopamine and oxytocin interactions underlying behaviors: Potential contributions to behavioral disorders *CNS Neuroscience & Therapeutics* **16** e92-123

[16] Baskerville T A, Allard J, Wayman C and Douglas A J 2009 Dopamine–oxytocin interactions in penile erection *European Journal of Neuroscience* **30** 2151-64

[17] Shapiro L E and Insel T R 1989 Ontogeny of oxytocin receptors in rat forebrain: A quantitative study *Synapse* **4** 259-66

[18] Krol K M, Moulder R G, Lillard T S, Grossmann T and Connelly J J 2019 Epigenetic dynamics in infancy and the impact of maternal engagement *Science Advances* **5** eaay0680

[19] LeClerc S and Easley D 2015 Pharmacological therapies for autism spectrum disorder: A review *P T* **40** 389-97

[20] Modahl C, Fein D, Waterhouse L and Newton N 1992 Does oxytocin deficiency mediate social deficits in autism? *J Autism Dev Disord* **22** 449-51

[21] Modahl C, Green L A, Fein D, Morris M, Waterhouse L, Feinstein C and Levin H 1998 Plasma oxytocin levels in autistic children *Biological Psychiatry* **43** 270-7

[22] Parker K J, Oztan O, Libove R A, Sumiyoshi R D, Jackson L P, Karhson D S, Summers J E, Hinman K E, Motonaga K S, Phillips J M, Carson D S, Garner J P and Hardan A Y 2017 Intranasal oxytocin treatment for social deficits and biomarkers of response in children with autism *Proc Natl Acad Sci USA* **114** 8119-24

[23] Green L, Fein D, Modahl C, Feinstein C, Waterhouse L and Morris M 2001 Oxytocin and autistic disorder: Alterations in peptide forms *Biological Psychiatry* **50** 609-13

[24] Andari E, Duhamel J-R, Zalla T, Herbrecht E, Leboyer M and Sirigu A 2010 Promoting social behavior with oxytocin in high-functioning autism spectrum disorders *PNAS* **107** 4389-94

[25] Guastella A J, Einfeld S L, Gray K M, Rinehart N J, Tonge B J, Lambert T J and Hickie I B 2010 Intranasal oxytocin improves emotion recognition for youth with autism spectrum disorders *Biological Psychiatry* **67** 692-4

[26] Tachibana M, Kagitani-Shimono K, Mohri I, Yamamoto T, Sanefuji W, Nakamura A, Oishi M, Kimura T, Onaka T, Ozono K and Taniike M 2013 Long-term administration of intranasal oxytocin is a safe and promising therapy for early adolescent boys with autism spectrum disorders *Journal of Child and Adolescent Psychopharmacology* **23** 123-7

[27] Anagnostou E, Soorya L, Brian J, Dupuis A, Mankad D, Smile S and Jacob S 2014 Intranasal oxytocin in the treatment of autism spectrum disorders: A review of literature and early safety and efficacy data in youth *Brain Research* **1580** 188-98

[28] Dadds M R, MacDonald E, Cauchi A, Williams K, Levy F and Brennan J 2014 Nasal oxytocin for social deficits in childhood autism: A randomized controlled trial *J Autism Dev Disord* **44** 521-31

[29] Guastella A J, Gray K M, Rinehart N J, Alvares G A, Tonge B J, Hickie I B, Keating C M, Cacciotti-Saija C and Einfeld S L 2015 The effects of a course of intranasal oxytocin on social behaviors in youth diagnosed with autism spectrum disorders: A randomized controlled trial *Journal of Child Psychology and Psychiatry* **56** 444-52

[30] Yatawara C J, Einfeld S L, Hickie I B, Davenport T A and Guastella A J 2016 The effect of oxytocin nasal spray on social interaction deficits observed in young children with autism: A randomized clinical crossover trial *Molecular Psychiatry* **21** 1225-31

[31] Strathearn L, Kim S, Bastian D A, Jung J, Iyengar U, Martinez S, Goin-Kochel R P and Fonagy P 2018 Visual systemizing preference in children with autism: A randomized controlled trial of intranasal oxytocin *Development and Psychopathology* **30** 511-21

[32] Ooi Y P, Weng S-J, Kossowsky J, Gerger H and Sung M 2017 Oxytocin and autism spectrum disorders: A systematic review and meta-analysis of randomized controlled trials *Pharmacopsychiatry* **50** 5-13

[33] Baron-Cohen S, Wheelwright S, Hill J, Raste Y and Plumb I 2001 The "Reading the Mind in the Eyes" Test revised version: A study with normal adults, and adults with asperger

syndrome or high-functioning autism *Journal of Child Psychology and Psychiatry* **42** 241-51

[34] Lord C, Risi S, Lambrecht L, Cook E H, Leventhal B L, DiLavore P C, Pickles A and Rutter M 2000 The Autism Diagnostic Observation Schedule-Generic: A standard measure of social and communication deficits associated with the spectrum of autism *J Autism Dev Disord* **30** 205-23

[35] Aman M G, Singh N N, Stewart A W and Field C J 1985 The aberrant behavior checklist: A behavior rating scale for the assessment of treatment effects *Am J Ment Defic* **89** 485-91

[36] Achenbach T M and Edelbrock C 1991 Child behavior checklist *Burlington (Vt)* **7** 371-92

[37] Constantino J N and Gruber C P 2005 *Social Responsiveness Scale* (WPS)

[38] Reynolds C R and Kamphaus R W 1992 *Behavior Assessment System for Children* (Circle Pines, MN: American Guidance Service)

[39] Wolf J M, Tanaka J W, Klaiman C, Cockburn J, Herlihy L, Brown C, South M, McPartland J, Kaiser M D, Phillips R and Schultz R T 2008 Specific impairment of face processing abilities in children with autism spectrum disorder using the Let's Face It! Skills Battery *Autism Res* **1** 329-40

[40] Dennis M, Purvis K, Barnes M A, Wilkinson M and Winner E 2001 Understanding of literal truth, ironic criticism, and deceptive praise following childhood head injury *Brain and Language* **78** 1-16

[41] Happé F G E 1994 An advanced test of theory of mind: Understanding of story characters' thoughts and feelings by able autistic, mentally handicapped, and normal children and adults *J Autism Dev Disord* **24** 129-54

[42] Gadow K and Sprafkin J 2009 *The symptom inventories: An annotated bibliography*

[43] Bodfish J W, Symons F J, Parker D E and Lewis M H 2000 Varieties of repetitive behavior in autism: Comparisons to mental retardation *J Autism Dev Disord* **30** 237-43

[44] Scahill L, Riddle M A, McSwiggin-Hardin M, Ort S I, King R A, Goodman W K, Cicchetti D and Leckman J F 1997 Children's Yale-Brown obsessive compulsive scale: Reliability and validity *Journal of the American Academy of Child & Adolescent Psychiatry* **36** 9

[45] Baron-Cohen S 2007 *Mind reading: The interactive guide to emotions* (Jessica Kingsley Publishers)

[46] Gresham F M and Elliott S N 1990 *The Social Skills Rating System* (American Guidance Service)

[47] Tonge B J, Brereton A V, Gray K M and Einfeld S L 1999 Behavioural and emotional disturbance in high-functioning autism and asperger syndrome *Autism* **3** 117-30

[48] Nowicki S and Duke M P 2001 Nonverbal receptivity: The Diagnostic Analysis of Nonverbal Accuracy (DANVA) *Interpersonal sensitivity: Theory and measurement* The LEA series in personality and clinical psychology (Mahwah, NJ, US: Lawrence Erlbaum Associates Publishers) pp 183-98

[49] Moore D G, Hobson R P and Lee A 1997 Components of person perception: An investigation with autistic, non-autistic retarded and typically developing children and adolescents *British Journal of Developmental Psychology* **15** 401-23

[50] Einfeld S L and Tonge B J 1995 The Developmental Behavior Checklist: The development and validation of an instrument to assess behavioral and emotional disturbance in children and

adolescents with mental retardation *J Autism Dev Disord* **25** 81-104

[51] Guy W 1976 *ECDEU assessment manual for psychopharmacology* (Rockville, Md: U.S. Dept. of Health, Education, and Welfare, Public Health Service, Alcohol, Drug Abuse, and Mental Health Administration, National Institute of Mental Health, Psychopharmacology Research Branch, Division of Extramural Research Programs)

[52] Brannan A M, Heflinger C A and Bickman L 1997 The caregiver strain questionnaire: Measuring the impact on the family of living with a child with serious emotional disturbance *Journal of Emotional and Behavioral Disorders* **5** 212-22

[53] Spence S H, Barrett P M and Turner C M 2003 Psychometric properties of the Spence Children's Anxiety Scale with young adolescents *Journal of Anxiety Disorders* **17** 605-25

[54] Gordon I, Wyk B C V, Bennett R H, Cordeaux C, Lucas M V, Eilbott J A, Zagoory-Sharon O, Leckman J F, Feldman R and Pelphrey K A 2013 Oxytocin enhances brain function in children with autism *PNAS* **110** 20953-8

[55] Gordon I, Jack A, Pretzsch C M, Vander Wyk B, Leckman J F, Feldman R and Pelphrey K A 2016 Intranasal oxytocin enhances connectivity in the neural circuitry supporting social motivation and social perception in children with autism *Sci Rep* **6** 35054

[56] Greene R K, Spanos M, Alderman C, Walsh E, Bizzell J, Mosner M G, Kinard J L, Stuber G D, Chandrasekhar T, Politte L C, Sikich L and Dichter G S 2018 The effects of intranasal oxytocin on reward circuitry responses in children with autism spectrum disorder *Journal of Neurodevelopmental Disorders* **10** 12

[57] Baker E and Stavropoulos K K M 2020 The effects of oxytocin administration on individuals with ASD: Neuroimaging and behavioral evidence *Progress in Molecular Biology and Translational Science* Autism vol 173, ed M Ilieva and W K W Lau (Elsevier) pp 209-38

[58] Eldevik S, Hastings R P, Hughes J C, Jahr E, Eikeseth S and Cross S 2009 Meta-analysis of early intensive behavioral intervention for children with autism *Journal of Clinical Child & Adolescent Psychology* **38** 439-50

[59] Kasari C and Lawton K 2010 New directions in behavioral treatment of autism spectrum disorders *Curr Opin Neurol* **23** 137-43

[60] Dawson G, Rogers S, Munson J, Smith M, Winter J, Greenson J, Donaldson A and Varley J 2010 Randomized, controlled trial of an intervention for toddlers with autism: The Early Start Denver Model *Pediatrics* **125** e17-23

[61] Reichow B, Barton E E, Boyd B A and Hume K 2012 Early intensive behavioral intervention (EIBI) for young children with autism spectrum disorders (ASD) *Cochrane Database Syst Rev* **10** CD009260

[62] Howlin P, Magiati I, Charman T and MacLean J 2009 Systematic review of early intensive behavioral interventions for children with autism *Am J Intellect Dev Disabil* **114** 23-41

[63] Dawson G and Burner K 2011 Behavioral interventions in children and adolescents with autism spectrum disorder: A review of recent findings *Curr Opin Pediatr* **23** 616-20

[64] Schreibman L, Dawson G, Stahmer A C, Landa R, Rogers S J, McGee G G, Kasari C, Ingersoll B, Kaiser A P, Bruinsma Y, McNerney E, Wetherby A and Halladay A 2015 Naturalistic developmental behavioral interventions: Empirically validated treatments for autism spectrum disorder *J Autism Dev Disord* **45** 2411-28

[65] Hart B M and Risley T R 1968 Establishing use of descriptive adjectives in the spontaneous speech of disadvantaged preschool children *J Appl Behav Anal* **1** 109-20

[66] Ingersoll B 2010 Brief report: Pilot randomized controlled trial of reciprocal imitation training for teaching elicited and spontaneous imitation to children with autism *J Autism Dev Disord* **40** 1154-60

[67] Ingersoll B and Schreibman L 2006 Teaching reciprocal imitation skills to young children with autism using a naturalistic behavioral approach: Effects on language, pretend play, and joint attention *J Autism Dev Disord* **36** 487-505

[68] Ingersoll B and Wainer A 2013 Initial efficacy of Project ImPACT: A parent-mediated social communication intervention for young children with asd *J Autism Dev Disord* **43** 2943-52

[69] Kasari C, Freeman S and Paparella T 2006 Joint attention and symbolic play in young children with autism: a randomized controlled intervention study *J Child Psychol Psychiatry* **47** 611-20

[70] Kasari C, Paparella T, Freeman S and Jahromi L B 2008 Language outcome in autism: Randomized comparison of joint attention and play interventions *Journal of Consulting and Clinical Psychology* **76** 125

[71] Rogers S J and Dawson G 2009 *Early start denver model curriculum checklist for young children with autism* (Guilford Press)

[72] Fuller E A, Oliver K, Vejnoska S F and Rogers S J 2020 The effects of the Early Start Denver Model for children with autism spectrum disorder: A meta-analysis *Brain Sciences* **10** 368

[73] Koegel R L and Koegel L K 2006 *Pivotal response treatments for autism: Communication, social, & academic development* (Baltimore, MD, US: Paul H Brookes Publishing)

[74] Koegel R L, Koegel L K and Carter C M 1999 Pivotal teaching interactions for children with autism *School Psychology Review* **28** 576-94

[75] Koegel R L, Koegel L K and McNerney E K 2001 Pivotal areas in intervention for autism *Journal of Clinical Child & Adolescent Psychology* **30** 19-32

[76] Verschuur R, Didden R, Lang R, Sigafoos J and Huskens B 2014 Pivotal response treatment for children with autism spectrum disorders: A systematic review *Rev J Autism Dev Disord* **1** 34-61

[77] Bozkus-Genc G and Yucesoy-Ozkan S 2016 Meta-analysis of pivotal response training for children with autism spectrum disorder *Education and Training in Autism and Developmental Disabilities* **51** 13-26

[78] Stavropoulos K K M 2017 Using neuroscience as an outcome measure for behavioral interventions in autism spectrum disorders (ASD): A review *Research in Autism Spectrum Disorders* **35** 62-73

[79] Dawson G, Jones E J H, Merkle K, Venema K, Lowy R, Faja S, Kamara D, Murias M, Greenson J, Winter J, Smith M, Rogers S J and Webb S J 2012 Early behavioral intervention is associated with normalized brain activity in young children with autism *J Am Acad Child Adolesc Psychiatry* **51** 1150-9

[80] Voos A C, Pelphrey K A, Tirrell J, Bolling D Z, Vander Wyk B, Kaiser M D, McPartland J C, Volkmar F R and Ventola P 2013 Neural mechanisms of improvements in social motivation after pivotal response treatment: two case studies *J Autism Dev Disord* **43** 1-10

[81] Kaiser M D, Hudac C M, Shultz S, Lee S M, Cheung C, Berken A M, Deen B, Pitskel N B, Sugrue D R, Voos A

C, Saulnier C A, Ventola P, Wolf J M, Klin A, Vander Wyk B C and Pelphrey K A 2010 Neural signatures of autism *Proc Natl Acad Sci U S A* **107** 21223-8

[82] Ventola P, Yang D Y J, Friedman H E, Oosting D, Wolf J, Sukhodolsky D G and Pelphrey K A 2015 Heterogeneity of neural mechanisms of response to pivotal response treatment *Brain Imaging Behav* **9** 74-88

[83] Van Hecke A V, Stevens S, Carson A M, Karst J S, Dolan B, Schohl K, McKindles R J, Remmel R and Brockman S 2015 Measuring the plasticity of social approach: A randomized controlled trial of the effects of the PEERS intervention on EEG asymmetry in adolescents with autism spectrum disorders *Journal of Autism and Developmental Disorders* **45** 316-35

[84] Laugeson E A and Frankel F 2011 *Social skills for teenagers with developmental and autism spectrum disorders: The PEERS treatment manual* (Routledge)

[85] Laugeson E A, Frankel F, Gantman A, Dillon A R and Mogil C 2012 Evidence-based social skills training for adolescents with autism spectrum disorders: The UCLA PEERS program *J Autism Dev Disord* **42** 1025-36

[86] Laugeson E A, Frankel F, Mogil C and Dillon A R 2009 Parent-assisted social skills training to improve friendships in teens with autism spectrum disorders *J Autism Dev Disord* **39** 596-606

[87] Mitchell A M and Pössel P 2012 Frontal brain activity pattern predicts depression in adolescent boys *Biological Psychology* **89** 525-7

[88] Venkataraman A, Yang D Y J, Dvornek N, Staib L H, Duncan J S, Pelphrey K A and Ventola P 2016 Pivotal response treatment prompts a functional rewiring of the brain among individuals with autism spectrum disorder *Neuroreport* **27** 1081-5

[89] Yang D, Pelphrey K A, Sukhodolsky D G, Crowley M J, Dayan E, Dvornek N C, Venkataraman A, Duncan J, Staib L and Ventola P 2016 Brain responses to biological motion predict treatment outcome in young children with autism *Transl Psychiatry* **6** e948

[90] Baker E, Veytsman E, Martin A M, Blacher J and Stavropoulos K K M 2020 Increased neural reward responsivity in adolescents with ASD after social skills intervention *Brain Sciences* **10** 402

[91] Constantino J N 2012 *Social Responsiveness Scale* (WPS)

[92] Gresham F M and Elliott S N 2008 *Social Skills Improvement System Rating Scales* (Pearson)

[93] Spanos M, Chandrasekhar T, Kim S-J, Hamer R M, King B H, McDougle C J, Sanders K B, Gregory S G, Kolevzon A, Veenstra-VanderWeele J and Sikich L 2020 Rationale, design, and methods of the Autism Centers of Excellence (ACE) network Study of Oxytocin in Autism to improve Reciprocal Social Behaviors (SOARS-B) *Contemp Clin Trials* **98** 106103

[94] Webb S J, Jones E J H, Kelly J and Dawson G 2014 The motivation for very early intervention for infants at high risk for autism spectrum disorders *International Journal of Speech-Language Pathology* **16** 36-42

[95] Zachor D and Ben-Itzchak E 2017 Variables affecting outcome of early intervention in autism spectrum disorder *J Pediatr Neurol* **15** 129-33

[96] Eldevik S, Hastings R P, Jahr E and Hughes J C 2012 Outcomes of behavioral intervention for children with autism in mainstream pre-school settings *J Autism Dev Disord* **42** 210-20

Chapter 6

Regulation of Morphological and Functional Aspects of Sexual Dimorphism in the Brain

Chitose Orikasa

Abstract

Sexual dimorphism of the adult brain regulates sex-dependent functions including reproductive and neuroendocrine activities in rodents. It is determined by sex steroid hormones during a critical perinatal period in female and male rodents. Sex steroids act on each nuclear receptor in the brain and control different physiological and neuroendocrine functions and behaviors. Several regions of the brain show evident morphological sex differences that are involved in their physiological functions. This review addresses and focuses largely on the role of sex-dependent differences in the brain, and their crucial functions in animal models. Particularly, recent intriguing data concerning the diversity of neuronal functions and sexual dimorphism are discussed.

Keywords: Sexual dimorphism, Sex steroid: Estrogen, ERα, ERβ, Neuronal plasticity

1. Introduction

Sexual dimorphism is characterized by morphological and physiological changes driven by sex steroids. In the rodent brain, it occurs during a critical period characterized by higher plasticity of neurons allowing changes in neuronal circuits and connectivity. For instance, hormonal manipulation during this time window, such as castration in males or replacement therapy in females (injections of androgen or estrogen), resulted in the conversion of intrinsic features and alteration of structures and functions of neural circuits in the brain. In rodents, critical time span for brain sex differentiation extends from embryonic day (ED) 18 to the postnatal day 10 [1], while in human it is exclusively embryonic day (ED12–22). Post this critical period, neuronal plasticity is lost and the effects of sex steroids can be diverted to activational effects in the brain. The mechanisms involved in defining the timing and duration of the neonatal critical period for the brain sexual differentiation remains to be determined. It is proposed that epigenetic modifications such as DNA methylation and histone acetylation might control the expression of genes implicated in brain sexual dimorphism [2].

The neuroendocrine systems, which control the action of sex steroids, including that on neural circuits, are differentiated in a sex-dependent manner, resulting in the regulation of reproductive and sex-specific behaviors. The actions of sex steroids in masculinization and feminization of the brain are mediated by steroid hormone receptors. In both human and nonhuman primates, young male and females show sex differences in toy preferences [3, 4]. Girls with congenital adrenal hyperplasia (CAH) show to preference toward toys of males and to have decreased female-typical behavior [5]. These results argue that behavioral sex differences are caused by sex steroids. Estrogen is produced locally in the brain from testosterone by the aromatase cytochrome P450 enzyme [6, 7] and affects sexual differentiation by biding to estrogen receptor (ER) in rodents. Maternal and fetal estrogen can be bound by the α-fetoprotein produced by fetal liver cells and yolk-sac cells, thereby preventing their passage through the blood–brain barrier [8]. This mechanism results in female brain being free from estrogen. In contrast, in males, testosterone crosses the blood–brain barrier and is converted by aromatase to elicit sexual differentiation of the brain [6, 7, 9]. The effects of testosterone and its enzymatic derivative, estradiol, on their receptors are therefore critical for the sexual differentiation of the brain.

2. Region-specific regulation of the ER

2.1 Sex-specific differences in the anteroventral periventricular nucleus

The crucial role of estrogens in the sexual differentiation of the brain is mediated by estrogen receptors subtypes ERα [10, 11] and ERβ [12]. The amount of steroid hormone receptors differentiated and available development differs between sexes. The anteroventral periventricular nucleus (AVPV) is greater in size and cell number in females than in males [13, 14]. In the AVPV, the distribution of ERα is similar in both sexes, but its expression levels are higher in females than in males in prepubertal and adult rats [15]. In contrast, the distribution pattern for ERβ detected by nonisotopic *in situ* hybridization and immunohistochemistry is different between sexes [16]. Specifically, in females, a vast majority of ERβ-positive cells is located in the most medial portion of the AVPV, whereas the ERβ-containing cells in males are dispersed more laterally in the AVPV (**Figure 1**). The distribution of ERβ is reversed by neonatal hormonal manipulations [16]. Therefore, sex-specific physiological functions are predictable for sexual dimorphism in the AVPV.

2.2 ERβ sexual dimorphism in the AVPV

Steroid-mediated organization of the brain might involve cell apoptosis, cell migration, neurogenesis, cell differentiation and synaptogenesis. Estrogen and androgen induce programmed cell death [17] by the sequential activation of cysteine-dependent asparate-specific proteases (caspase) during the development of the hypothalamus [18] in the dimorphism of dopaminergic neurons in the AVPV [19–21]. The total number of ERβ-positive cells within the AVPV is not different between intact females and males [15, 22]. This is assumed to be caused by mechanisms other than apoptosis namely the sexual dimorphic expression of ERβ in the AVPV. The sexual dimorphic features of the brain caused by sex steroids do not always coincide with larger nuclei exclusively in one sex. Indeed, a region-specific ERβ gene expression is observed in the AVPV [22]. Moreover, the steroids might act on specific regions in the brain [22]. In brain slices from developing mouse brain, estradiol but not dihydrotestosterone induces and modulates neuronal migration [23, 24]. These results suggest that sexual dimorphism of ERβ in the AVPV might contribute to migration rather than apoptosis or neurogenesis.

2.3 Functional implications in ERα and ERβ localization in the AVPV

In the AVPV of female rats, a majority of ERβ-positive cells also express ERα [16]. It has been shown that ERα together with kisspeptin regulates ovulation, while ERβ is

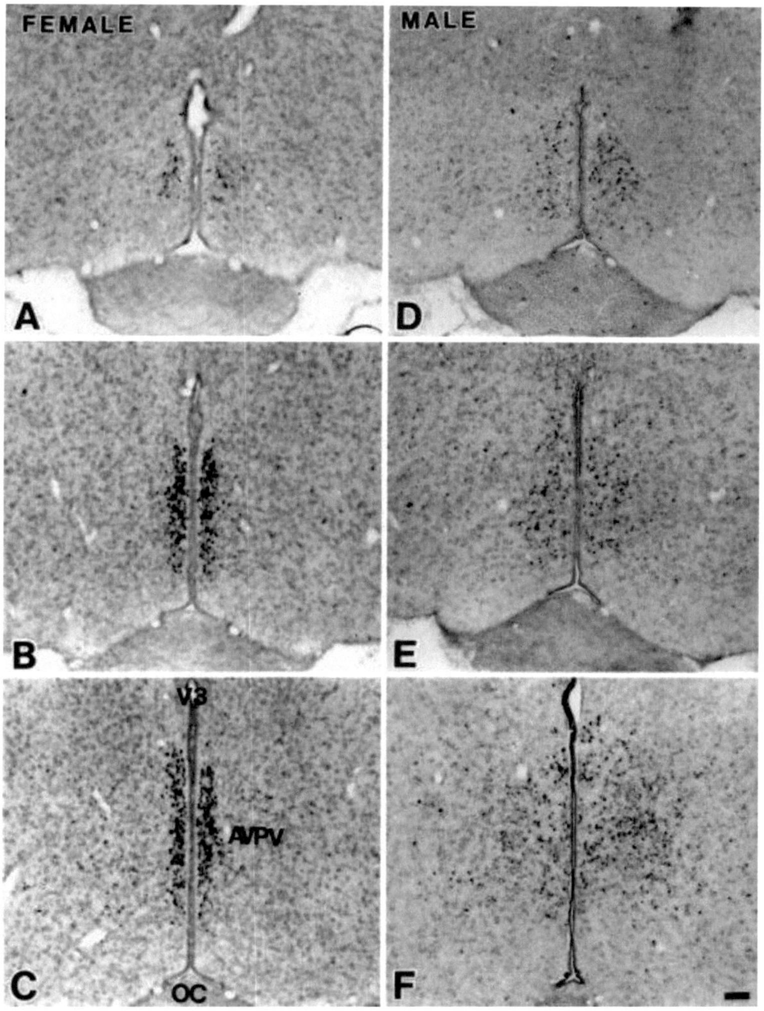

Figure 1.
Sexual dimorphism in the AVPV. ERβ positive cells aggregated densely in females (A-C), whereas the ERβ-containing cells in males (D-F) dispersed more laterally in the AVPV in the AVPV. Scale, 100 μm. From [16].

rather modified by these events [25]. At the molecular level, ERs bind to an estrogen responsive element (ERE) [26] after heterodimer formation [27], which allows the integration and collaboration of various signaling pathways for the completion of ovulation. The experimental infusion of antisense oligonucleotides in females results in decreased ERβ expression in the AVPV and consequently a persistent estrous [16]. Moreover, ERβ-positive cells and dopaminergic neurons have comparable distribution patterns in the AVPV [16]. Both ERα and ERβ have a role in the sexual dimorphism of dopaminergic neurons in the AVPV in both sexes [16, 28]. The secretion of luteinizing hormone (LH) is controlled by dopaminergic projections to neurons producing the gonadotropin-releasing hormone (GnRH) [29]. The cycle of female rats stalls ovulation state by small lesions of the AVPV [30]. Altogether, these data suggest that ERα and ERβ are colocalized with GnRH and are involved in LH secretion [31, 32]. In particular, ERα exerts a positive role for GnRH neurons, while ERβ exerts a negative control of those neurons [25]. Nonclassical ERE-independent ERα effects are involved in negative regulation on pulsatile GnRH secretion, while ERβ effects are involved in positive regulation on that secretion [31, 33]. It is still controversial to regulate GnRH neurons by ERs. Considering the inherent male distribution pattern of ERβ, a peculiar characteristic of the dopaminergic innervation in the AVPV [28] might be responsible for the GnRH secretion in the brain of males.

2.4 Formation of the sexually dimorphic nucleus in the preoptic area

The sexually dimorphic nucleus in the preoptic area (SDN-POA) was first characterized by Nissl staining, revealing in a larger volume in the brain of male rats than that in the brain of female rats [1, 34]. The volume of this nucleus is altered by gonadal steroids during the perinatal critical period [1]. Somatostatin might also be involved in sexual dimorphism in the SDN-POA. Indeed, during development, cells positive for somatostatin are expressed in a sex-dependent manner in the SDN-POA. Sex reversal of the dimorphism of somatostatin expression is observed in orchidectomized males and estrogen treated female pups [35]. The somatostatin mRNA-positive cells are significantly more in males than in females, but eventually the difference recedes. Somatostatin expression in females is steady during the postnatal development. The transcription of somatostatin is transient and seems to contribute to the development of the SDN-POA. Somatostatin might prompt neuronal differentiation and survival via the somatostatin receptor.

Immunostaining against calbindin D28k, a major cytoplasmic calcium-binding and buffering protein, has been successfully used to identify the rat hypothalamus [36], SDN-POA [35, 37] and provides an alternative to Nissl staining [37]. Distribution of calbindin-labeled cells in the SDN-POA is similar to somatostatin in both sexes. It has been suggested that apoptosis has a role in sexual differentiation of the SDN-POA [38]. However, no difference in the total numbers of calbindin positive cells was observed in the SDN-POA after perinatal administration of bromodeoxyuridine in both sexes [39]. On the contrary, in the postnatal SDN-POA, these neurons still show an aggregated distribution in females, while they are dispersed laterally in males [39]. Altogether, these data suggest that, besides apoptosis, cell proliferation and migration might contribute to the morphological difference in the rat SDN-POA. Moreover, ERα are reported to be expressed in the SDN-POA [40], suggesting the presence of estrogenic action in the SDN-POA sexual dimorphism.

Moreover, Nissl stained SDN-POA had not been reported in mouse until recently identified by calbindin immunohistochemistry [41] (**Figure 2**). The morphological sex-dependent differences of the mouse SDN-POA were first demonstrated and established in terms of morphology and linked to gonadal steroid hormones during the prenatal critical period. Male mice have a greater number of calbindin-positive cells than females [41]. Similar differences within medial POA/anterior hypothalamic area (AHA) are observed in sheep, which are smaller in females than in males [42]. The volume of this nucleus in males is smaller in male-oriented than in female-oriented individuals. In humans, interstitial nuclei of the anterior hypothalamus (INAH) are considered comparable to those of rodent and sheep. The INAH is smaller in females than in males and smaller in homosexual men than in heterosexual men [43]. These results suggested that the sexual dimorphic nucleus in the two species is involved in sexual orientation. The male mice copulatory behavior and the preference for females is attributed to this difference in the SDN-POA [44–47]. Further functional analysis is required to completely understand the mechanisms involved in the sexual dimorphism of the SDN-POA.

2.5 Sexual dimorphic expression and function of ERs in the preoptic area

In the preoptic area (POA), ERα expression is much higher in females than in males [48]. This sex difference occurs during the perinatal period. After birth, the

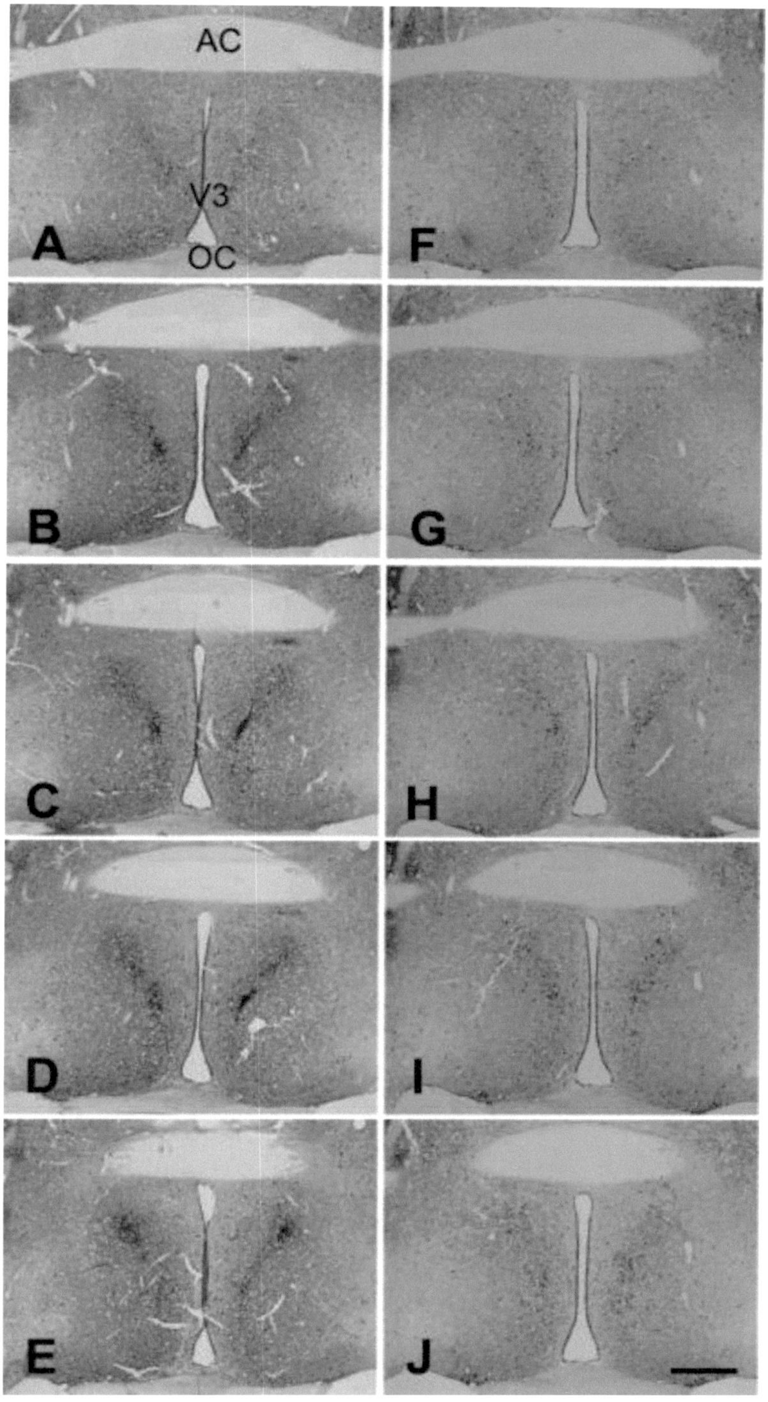

Figure 2.
Sexual dimorphism in the SDN-POA. Calbindin (CB)-immunoreactive cells in the mouse SDN-POA in males (A-E) and in females (F-J) in the rostral-caudal direction. In males (B-D), but not females, a cell aggregate of CB-positive cells is prominent. Sale, 400 µm. From [41].

expression of ERs is down regulated in the POA by estrogen [49]. The decreased ERα expression occurs in both sexes but the differential expression in the POA between females and males persists throughout life. Although the ERα levels are higher in females than in males, a comparable distribution pattern of ERα is observed [16, 48]. The POA has been implicated to be involved in steroid activation of the male copulatory behavior [50]. In particular, dopamine neurons in the mPOA prompt male sexual behavior [51]. ERα and oxytocin containing neurons in the mPOA participate to control copulatory behavior in male rats [52–54]. In females, the POA and the adjacent bed nucleus of the stria terminalis (BNST) is considered essential for controlling maternal [55–58] and mating behaviors [59]. ERα in the mPOA is involved in the regulation of maternal care, maternal aggression and sexual behavior [56]. ERβ is detected by *in situ* hybridization and immunohistochemistry in the medial preoptic nucleus (mPOA) and more caudally in the BNST [16] (**Figure 3**). In males, ERβ in the mPOA is involved in aggressive behavior [60]. Overall in rodents, identical brain regions control specific behaviors depending on the sex. Recently, it is shown that the male-typical mounting behavior and female-typical pup retrieval behavior are induced by ERα located in the same region of the POA [61]. These data suggest that the sex specific neural circuits are able to control opposite behaviors. Therefore, sex-typical behaviors are likely induced by the harmonic expression of sex specific receptors together with sex steroid. Besides the neural circuit with a high degree of plasticity in the sexual dimorphic nervous system assuring precise sex-specific behavior events, there may be a possible the involvement of circumstances in ensuring responsiveness of the sex steroids.

2.6 Functional diversity of the ventromedial hypothalamus

The volume of the ventromedial hypothalamus (VMH) is larger in males than in females [62, 63]. ERα and ERβ are expressed in the VMH of rodents [22, 48].

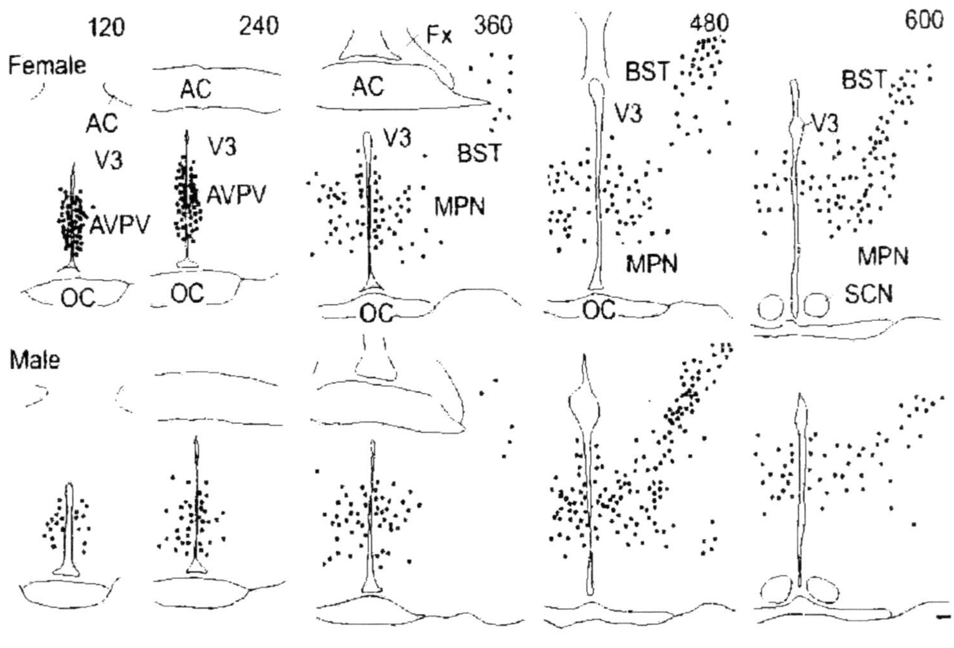

Figure 3.
Schematic representation of the distribution of ERβ mRNA-positive cells in the forebrain of rats through rostrocaudal axis. Scale, 100 μm. AC, anterior commissure; AVPV, anteroventral periventricular nucleus; BST, bed nucleus of the stria terminals; Fx, fornix; MPN, medial preoptic nucleus; OC, optic chiasm; SCN, suprachiasmatic nucleus; V3, third ventricle. From [16].

However, ERα expression is abundant in the ventrolateral portion of the VMH and is higher in female rats than in male rats [48]. The sex difference is most likely due to the conversion of testosterone into estrogen, which downregulates ERα expression. Moreover, the aromatase signal in males is more robust than in females [64]. A sex difference in ERβ expression is observed in both postnatal day 14 and in the adult rat brain, indicating that the sexual dimorphism is also maintained throughout life [22]. ERβ expression in the adult VMH is downregulated by estrogen or testosterone administration. The difference in expression is reversed by administration of estrogen in female rats or orchidectomy male rats. This sexual dimorphism is entirely attributable to the effects of sex steroids on the brain organization and plasticity during the critical neonatal period of the brain. Estrogen, converted from circulating androgen in males, downregulates ERα and ERβ expression in the VMH [22, 48] and consequently physiological functions. Estrogen together with progesterone in the VMH induces female sexual reproductive behavior such as lordosis, sexual receptivity and odor preference [65].

In adult males, the expression of ERα is lower than that in females. Cells in the male VMH are activated during fighting [66]. In these processes, ERα is involved in sexual [67] and aggressive behaviors in mice [68, 69], whereas ERβ is assume to be inhibitory to the aggressive behavior [68]. Other studies have demonstrated that male sexual behavior is not affected by ERβ in the VMH [70], but is profoundly regulated by ERα and the androgen receptor (AR), suggesting a possible distinct role for ERβ and ERα on each behavior. Opposing social behaviors, such as mounting and attack, are regulated by ERα [67] or progesterone receptor [71] cells located in discrete regions of the VMH. Sex steroid receptor expression in the VMH is induced by environmental hormonal milieu during the critical period and in turn controls the dynamic action of the sex hormones on sex-specific behavior in adults [66, 72]. These data suggest that males and females seem to exhibit identical neural circuits in the VMH, but the activated receptors might contribute to inducing the sex-typical behavior. The sex-specific neural circuit dictated by sex steroids could work in conjunction with estrogen-mediated ERs.

3. Alternative mechanism for sexual dimorphism in the medial amygdala

The medial amygdala (MeA) is larger volume in males than in females [73] and this difference is abolished after castration in males and androgen treatment in females [74]. In adults, the size and volume of neurons is modified by circulating androgen. After castration of adult male rats, the cell soma size in the posterodorsal MeA (MePD) is similar to the one observed in females [74]. However, the number of MeA neurons in both sexes is not affected by adult androgens [75]. Steroid hormones also influence the organization of the MePD during the neonatal period [76, 77] and its metabolite, estrogen, results in masculinization of the MePD. ERα and ERβ are abundantly expressed in the MePD [22, 48, 78, 79] where the aromatase enzyme is also detected [80, 81]. ERs mediate estrogen-induced modifications in the MePD associated with masculinization and male-specific behaviors [82]. However, the masculinization in the MePD in the adult brain is mostly driven by circulating androgen [82]. Both the action of ER [82] and AR [83] in the MePD on the size of neuronal somas and in the sexual behavior mostly occurs in the adults [82]. In adults, there is no sex-dependent difference in ER subtype and expression in the MePD, but there is a sexual dimorphic expression of ERβ but not ERα in newborns [84]. Neonatal hormonal manipulations could not reverse the sex differences in ERβ in both sexes, suggesting that ERβ-mediated estrogen actions are not involved in the sexual dimorphism in the MePD. Furthermore, ERβ is highly expressed in the

MePD of adult female and male rats and is not affected by gonadectomy or estrogen treatment in both sexes [22]. Therefore, the ERβ expression also acts independent of activity in this structure.

In the MePD, sexual dimorphism involves mechanisms distinct from other regions of the brain. The MePD receives inputs from the olfactory and pheromonal systems, suggesting a functional role of this structure in sex arousal and regulation of adult social behaviors, including mating, aggressive [85, 86], and territorial behavior [87]. Acquisition of mating stimuli induces Fos in the ERs in the MeA [88]. Finally, the mechanisms induced by the ERs in the MeA and those involved in sexual stimuli [89], gonadotropin secretion [90], ovulation [91] sex and courtship behaviors [87], onset of puberty [92], parenting, and reproduction [85, 89, 93] still remain to be identified.

4. Conclusion

Sexual dimorphism is characterized by morphological differences in several regions of the brain. Morphological sex differences in the POA/AHA and the INAH were revealed in sheep and human brains, which are assumed to be important for determining sexual orientation. Expression of the phenotypes i.e., behavioral sex differences, are suggested to be derived from morphological sex differences in the brain. However, the morphological sex differences are subtly evident in other human brain regions; hence, their association with functional sex differences in the human brain remains controversial. Consequently, CAH results in masculinized female brain, thereby leading to male-typical preferences, which are the congenital characteristics inherently caused by steroid and not acquired by learning. Striking sex differences in animal models contribute in establishing the mechanisms of sexual dimorphism in the brain of all living beings.

ER expression levels contribute substantially to the physiological and behavioral differences. However, the extent to which the amounts of ER control the development of sexual dimorphism remains to be clarified. Sex-specific neural circuits activated by sex steroids might contribute to the functional role of ERs activated by estrogens. Recently it was evidenced that a high neuronal plasticity rate in neural circuits is necessary to ensure precise sex-specific responsiveness to sex steroids. The mechanism involved in the regulating the local action of sex steroids remains to be elucidated. Particularly, the expression and regulation of genes implicated in sexual dimorphism must be investigated.

Acknowledgements

This work was supported, in part, by grants-in-aid for scientific research from the Japanese Ministry of Education, Science, Sports and Culture [19 K12738 (2019-2021)] (C.O.).

Declarations interest

None.

Author details

Chitose Orikasa
Department of Bioregulation, Institute for Advanced Medical Science,
Nippon Medical School, Kawasaki, Japan

*Address all correspondence to: orikasa@nms.ac.jp

References

[1] Gorski, R.A., 1968. Influence of age on the response to paranatal administration of a low dose of androgen. Endocrinology. 82, 1001-1004.

[2] Forger, *Philos Trans R Soc Lond B Biol Sci*. 2016;371(1688):20150114.

[3] Berenbaum, S.A., 1999. Effects of early androgens on sex-typed activities and interests in adolescents with congenital adrenal hyperplasia. Horm. Behav. 35, 102-110.

[4] Grabowska, A., 2017. Sex on the brain: Are gender-dependent structural and functional differences associated with behavior? J Neurosci Res. 95, 200-212.

[5] Spencer, D., Pasterski, V., A S Neufeld, S.A.N., Glover, V., Thomas G O'Connor, T.G., Hindmarsh, P.C., Ieuan A Hughes, I.A., Acerini,C.L., Melissa Hines, M., 2021. Prenatal androgen exposure and children's gender-typed behavior and toy and playmate preferences Horm Behav. 127, 104889.

[6] MacLusky, N.J., Philip, A., Hurlburt C, Naftolin F. Estrogen formation in the developing rat brain: sex differences in aromatase activity during early post-natal life. Psychoneuroendocrinology. 1985, 10, 355-361.

[7] McEwen, B.S., Lieberburg, I., Chapta,l C., Krey, L., 1977. Aromatization: important for sexual differentiation of the neonatal rat brain. Horrn. Behav. 9, 249-263.

[8] MacLusky, N.J., Lieberburg, I., McEwen, B.S., 1979. The development of estrogen receptor systems in the rat brain: perinatal development. Brain Res. 178, 129-142.

[9] MacLusky, N.J., Naftolin, F., 1981. Sexual differentiation of the central nervous system. Science. 211, 1294-1303.

[10] Green, S., Walter, P., Kumar, V., Krust, A., Bornert, J.M., Argos, P., Chambon, P., 1986. Human oestrogen receptor cDNA: sequence, expression and homology to v-erb-A. Nature. 320, 134-139.

[11] Koike, S., Sakai, M., Muramatsu, M., 1987. Molecular cloning and characterization of rat estrogen receptor cDNA. Nucleic Acids Res. 15, 2499-2513.

[12] Kuiper, G.G.J.M., Enmark, E. Pelto-Huikko, M. Nilsson, S., Gustaffsson J.-A. 1996. Cloning of a novel estrogen receptor expressed in rat prostate and ovary. Proc. Natl. Acad. Sci. USA. 93, 5925-5930.

[13] Davis, E.C., Shryne, J.E., Gorski, R.A., 1996. Structural sexual dimorphisms in the anteroventral periventricular nucleus of the rat hypothalamus are sensitive to gonadal steroids perinatally, but develop peripubertally. Neuroendocrinology. 63, 142-148.

[14] Simerly, R.B., 1998. Organization and regulation of sexually dimorphic neuroendocrine pathways. Behav. Brain Res. 92, 195-203.

[15] Kanaya, M., Morishita, M., Tsukahara S., 2018. Temporal Expression Patterns of Genes Related to Sex Steroid Action in Sexually Dimorphic Nuclei During Puberty. Front Endocrinol (Lausanne). 9, 213.

[16] Orikasa, C., Kondo, Y., Hayash,i S., McEwen, B.S., Sakuma, Y., 2002. Sexually dimorphic expression of estrogen receptor beta in the anteroventral periventricular nucleus of the rat preoptic area: implication in luteinizing hormone surge. Proc Natl Acad. Sci. U.S.A. 99, 3306-3311.

[17] Arai, Y., Murakami, S., Nishizuka, M., 1994. Androgen enhances neuronal degeneration in the developing preoptic area: apoptosis in the anteroventral periventricular nucleus (AVPvN-POA). Horm. Behav. 28, 313-319.

[18] Thompson, C.K., Brenowitz, E.A., 2008. Caspase inhibitor infusion protects an avian song control circuit from seasonal-like neurodegeneration. J. Neurosci. 28,7130-7136.

[19] Forger, N.G., 2006. Cell death and sexual differentiation of the nervous system. Neuroscience. 138, 929-938.

[20] Tsukahara, S., 2009. Sex differences and the roles of sex steroids in apoptosis of sexually dimorphic nuclei of the preoptic area in postnatal rats. J. Neuroendocrinol. 21, 370-376.

[21] Waters, E.M., Richard B Simerly, R.B., 2009. Estrogen induces caspase-dependent cell death during hypothalamic development. J. Neurosci. 29, 9714-9718.

[22] Orikasa, C., Sakuma, Y., 2004. Sex and region-specific regulation of oestrogen receptor beta in the rat hypothalamus. J. Neuroendocrinol. 16, 964-969.

[23] Henderson, R.G., Brown, A.E., Tobet, S.A., 1999. Sex differences in cell migration in the preoptic area / anterior hypothalamus of mice. J. Neurobiol. 41, 252-266.

[24] Knoll, J.G., Wolfe, C.A., Tobet, S.A., 2007. Estrogen modulates neuronal movements within the developing preoptic area-anterior hypothalamus. Eur. J. Neurosci. 26, 1091-1099.

[25] Roa, J., Vigo, E., Castellano, J.M., Gaytan, F., Navarro, V.M., Aguilar, E., Dijcks, F.A. Ederveen, A.G.H., Pinilla, L., van Noort, P.I., Tena-Semper, M., 2008. Opposite roles of estrogen receptor (ER)-alpha and ERbeta in the modulation of luteinizing hormone responses to kisspeptin in the female rat: implications for the generation of the preovulatory surge. Endocrinology 149, 1627-1637.

[26] Li, X., Huang, J., Yi, P., Bambara, R.A., Hilf, R., Muyan, M., 2004. Single-chain estrogen receptors (ERs) reveal that the ERalpha/beta heterodimer emulates functions of the ERalpha dimer in genomic estrogen signaling pathways. Mol. Cell. Biol. 24, 7681-7694.

[27] Powell, E., Shanle, E., Brinkman, A., Li, J., Keles, S., Wisinski, K.B., Wei Huang, W., Xu W., 2012. Identification of estrogen receptor dimer selective ligands reveals growth-inhibitory effects on cells that co-express ERα and ERβ. PLoS One 7, e30993.

[28] Simerly, R.B., Zee, M.C., Pendleton, J.W., Lubahn, D.B., Korach, K.S., 1997. Estrogen receptor-dependent sexual differentiation of dopaminergic neurons in the preoptic region of the mouse. Proc. Natl. Acad. Sci. U.S.A. 94, 14077-14082.

[29] Cruz, M. E., Villegas, G., Dominguez-Gonzalez, A., Chavira, R. & Dominguez,R. (2001) *Brain Res. Bull.* **54,** 339-344.

[30] Wiegand, S. J., Terasawa, E. & Bridson, W. E. (1978) Endocrinology 102, 1645-1648.

[31] Hu, L., Gustofson, R.L., Feng, H., Leung, P.K., Mores, N., Krsmanovic, L.Z., Catt, K.J., 2008. Converse regulatory functions of estrogen receptor-alpha and -beta subtypes expressed in hypothalamic gonadotropin-releasing hormone neurons. Mol. Endocrinol. 22, 2250-2259.

[32] Skynner, M.J., Sim, J.A., Herbison, A.E., 1999. Detection of estrogen receptor a and b messenger ribonucleic

acids in adult gonadotropin-releasing hormone neurons. Endocrinology. 140, 5195-5201.

[33] Glidewell-Kenney, C., Hurley, L.A., Pfaff, L, Weiss, J., Levine, J.E., Jameson, J.L., 2007. Nonclassical estrogen receptor alpha signaling mediates negative feedback in the female mouse reproductive axis. Proc. Natl. Acad. Sci. U.S.A. 104, 198173-198177.

[34] Gorski, R.A., Harlan, R.E., Jacobson, C.D., Shryne, J.E. and Southam, A.M., 1980. Evidence for the existence of a sexually dimorphic nucleus in the preoptic area of the rat. J. Comp. Neurol. 193, 529-539.

[35] Orikasa, C., Kondo, Y., Sakuma, Y., 2007. Transient transcription of the somatostatin gene at the time of estrogen-dependent organization of the sexually dimorphic nucleus of the rat preoptic area. Endocrinology 148,1144-1149.

[36] Brager, D.H., Sickel, M.J., McCarthy, M.M., 2000. Developmental sex differences in calbindin-D(28K) and calretinin immunoreactivity in the neonatal rat hypothalamus. J. Neurobiol. 42, 315-322.

[37] Sickel, M.J., McCarthy, M.M., 2000. Calbindin-D28k immunoreactivity is a marker for a subdivision of the sexually dimorphic nucleus of the preoptic area of the rat: developmental profile and gonadal steroid modulation. J. Neuroendocrinol. 12, 397-402.

[38] Yang, S.L., Chen, Y.Y., Hsieh, Y.L., Jin, S.H., Hsu, H.K., Hsu, C. 2004. Perinatal androgenization prevents age-related neuron loss in the sexually dimorphic nucleus of the preoptic area in female rats. Dev. Neurosci. 26, 54-60.

[39] Orikasa, C., Kondo, Y., Usui, S., Sakuma, Y., 2010. Similar numbers of neurons are generated in the male and female rat preoptic area in utero. Neurosci. Res. 68, 9-14.

[40] Jeong, J.K., Ryu, B.J., Choi, J., Kim,D.H., Choi, E.J., Park, J.W., Park, J.J., Lee, B.J., 2008. NELL2 participates in formation of the sexually dimorphic nucleus of the pre-optic area in rats. J. Neurochem. 106, 1604-1613.

[41] Orikasa, C., Sakuma, Y., 2010. Estrogen configures sexual dimorphism in the preoptic area of C57BL/6J and ddN strains of mice. J. Comp. Neurol. 2010. 518, 3618-3629.

[42] Roselli, C.E., Larkin, K., Resko, J.A., Stellflug, J.N., Stormshak, F., 2004. The volume of a sexually dimorphic nucleus in the ovine medial preoptic area/ anterior hypothalamus varies with sexual partner preference. Endocrinology. 145, 478-483

[43] LeVay, S. 1991. A difference in hypothalamic structure between heterosexual and homosexual men. Science. 253, 1034-1037.

[44] Anderson, R.H., Fleming, D.E., Rhees, R.W., Kinghorn, E., 1986. Relationships between sexual activity, plasma testosterone, and the volume of the sexually dimorphic nucleus of the preoptic area in prenatally stressed and non-stressed rats. Brain Res. 370, 1-10.

[45] Hay-Schmidt, A., Finkielman, O.T.E., Jensen, B.A.H., Høgsbro , C.F., Holm, J.B., Johansen, K.H., Jense, T.K., 2017. Prenatal exposure to paracetamol/ acetaminophen and precursor aniline impairs masculinisation of male brain and behaviour. Reproduction. 154, 145-152.

[46] Houtsmuller, E.J., Brand, T., de Jonge, F.H., Joosten, R.N., van de Poll, N.E., Slob, A.K., 1994. SDN-POA volume, sexual behavior, and partner preference of male rats affected by perinatal treatment with ATD. Physiol. Behav. 56, 535-541.

[47] Rhees, R.W., Al-Saleh, H.N., Kinghorn, E.W., Fleming, D.E., Lephart, E.D., 1999. Relationship between sexual behavior and sexually dimorphic structures in the anterior hypothalamus in control and prenatally stressed male rats. Brain Res. Bull. 50, 193-199.

[48] Yokosuka, M., Okamura, H., Hayash,i S. 1997. Postnatal development and sex difference in neurons containing estrogen receptor-alpha immunoreactivity in the preoptic brain, the diencephalon, and the amygdala in the rat. J. Comp. Neurol. 389, 81-93.

[49] DonCarlos, L.L., McAbee, M., Ramer-Quinn, D.S., Stancik, D.M., 1995. Estrogen receptor mRNA levels in the preoptic area of neonatal rats are responsive to hormone manipulation. Developmental Bram Research. 84, 253-260.

[50] Kondo, Y., Arai, Y., 1995. Functional association between the medial amygdala and the medial preoptic area in regulation of mating behavior in the male rat. Physiol. Behav.57, 69-73.

[51] Dominguez, J.M., Gil, M., Hull, E.M., 2006. Preoptic glutamate facilitates male sexual behavior. J. Neurosci. 26, 1699-1703.

[52] Clancy, N., D Zumpe, D., Michael, R.P., 2000. Estrogen in the medial preoptic area of male rats facilitates copulatory behavior. Horm. Behav. 38, 86-93.

[53] Gil, M., Renu Bhatt, R., Picotte, K.B., Hull, E.M., 2013. Sexual experience increases oxytocin receptor gene expression and protein in the medial preoptic area of the male rat. Psychoneuroendocrinology. 38, 1688-1697.

[54] Panzica, G.C., Viglietti-Panzica, C., Balthazart, J., 1996 The sexually dimorphic medial preoptic nucleus of quail: a key brain area mediating steroid action on male sexual behavior. Front Neuroendocrinol. 17, 51-125.

[55] Numan, M., Stolzenberg, D.S., 2009. Medial preoptic area interactions with dopamine neural systems in the control of the onset and maintenance of maternal behavior in rats. Front. Neuroendocrin. 30, 46-64.

[56] Ribeiro, A.C., Musatov, S., Shteyler, A., Simanduyev, S., Arrieta-Cruz, I., Ogawa, S., Pfaff, D.W., 2012. siRNA silencing of estrogen receptor-α expression specifically in medial preoptic area neurons abolishes maternal care in female mice. Proc. Natl. Acad. Sci. U.S.A. 109, 16324-16329.

[57] Tsuneoka, Y, Maruyama T, Yoshida S, Nishimori K, Kato T, Numan M, Kuroda KO. Functional, anatomical, and neurochemical differentiation of medial preoptic area subregions in relation to maternal behavior in the mouse. J Comp Neurol. 2013 May 1;521(7):1633-1663.

[58] Wu, Z., Autry, A.E., Bergan, J.F., Watabe-Uchida, M., Dulac, C.G., 2014. Galanin neurons in the medial preoptic area govern parental behaviour. Nature. 509, 325-330.

[59] McHenry, J.A, Otis, J.M., Rossi, M.A., Robinson, J.E., Kosyk, O., Miller, N.W., McElligott, Z.A., Budygin, E.A., Rubinow, D.R., Stuber, G.D., 2017. Hormonal gain control of a medial preoptic area social reward circuit. Nat. Neurosci. 20, 449-458.

[60] Nakata, M., Sano, K., Musatov, S., Yamaguchi, N., Sakamoto, T., Ogawa, S., 2016. .Effects of Prepubertal or Adult Site-Specific Knockdown of Estrogen Receptor beta in the Medial Preoptic Area and Medial Amygdala on Social Behaviors in Male Mice. eNeuro. 3, ENEURO.0155-15.2016.

[61] Wei, Y.-C., Wang, S.-R., Jiao, Z.-L., Zhang, W., Lin, J.-K., Li, X.-Y., Li, S.-S.,

Xin Zhang, Xu, X.-H., 2018. Medial preoptic area in mice is capable of mediating sexually dimorphic behaviors regardless of gender. Nat. Commun. 9, 279.

[62] Madeira, M.D., Ferreira-Silva, L., Paula-Barbosa, M.M., 2001. Influence of sex and estrus cycle on the sexual dimorphisms of the hypothalamic ventromedial nucleus: stereological evaluation and Golgi study. J. Comp. Neurol. 432, 329-345.

[63] Matsumoto, A., Arai, Y., 1983. Sex difference in volume of the ventromedial nucleus of the hypothalamus in the rat. Endocrinol. Jpn. 30, 277-280.

[64] Dugger, B.N., Morris, J. A., Cynthia L Jordan, C.L., Breedlove, S.M., 2007. Androgen receptors are required for full masculinization of the ventromedial hypothalamus (VMH) in rats. Horm. Behav. 51, 195-201.

[65] Robarts, D.W., Baum, M.J., 2006. Ventromedial hypothalamic nucleus lesions disrupt olfactory mate recognition and receptivity in female ferrets. Horm. Behav. 51, 104-113.

[66] Lin, D., 1, Maureen P Boyle, M.P., Dollar, P., Lee, H., E S Lein, E.S., 2011. Pietro Perona, David J Anderson Functional identification of an aggression locus in the mouse hypothalamus Nature. 470, 221-226.

[67] Lee, H., Kim, D.W., Remedios, R., Anthony, T.E., Chang, A., Madisen, L., Zeng, H., Anderson, D.J., 2014a. Scalable control of mounting and attack by Esr1+ neurons in the ventromedial hypothalamus. Nature. 509, 627-632. doi: 10.1038/nature13169.54 Hyosang Lee, 2014

[68] Ogawa, S., Chester, A.E., Hewitt, S.C., Walker, V.R., Gustafsson, J.A., Smithies, O., Korach, K.S., Pfaff, D.W., 2000. Abolition of male sexual behaviors in mice lacking estrogen receptors alpha and beta (alpha beta ERKO). Proc Natl Acad Sci U S A. 97, 14737-14741.

[69] Wersinger, S.R., Sannen, K., Villalba, C., Lubahn, D.B., Rissman, E.F., De Vries, G.J., 1997. Masculine sexual behavior is disrupted in male and female mice lacking a functional estrogen receptor alpha gene. Horm. Behav. 32, 176-183.

[70] Naulé, L., Marie-Luce, C., Parmentier, C., Martini, M., Albac, C., Trouillet, A.C., Keller, M., Hardin-Pouzet, H., Mhaouty-Kodja, S., 2016. Revisiting the neural role of estrogen receptor beta in male sexual behavior by conditional mutagenesis. Horm. Behav. 80, 1-9.

[71] Yang, C.F., Chiang, M.C., Gray, D.C., Prabhakaran, M., Alvarado, M., Juntti, S.A., Unger, E.K., James A Wells, J.A., Shah, N.M., 2013. Sexually dimorphic neurons in the ventromedial hypothalamus govern mating in both sexes and aggression in males. Cell. 153, 896-909.

[72] Kudwa, A.E., Harada, N., Honda, S.-I. Rissman, E. F., 2007. Effects of organisational oestradiol on adult immunoreactive oestrogen receptors (alpha and beta) in the male mouse brain. J. Neuroendocrinol. 19, 767-772.

[73] Hines M, Allen LS, Gorski RA (1992) Sex differences in subregions of the medial nucleus of the amygdala and the bed nucleus of the stria terminalis in the rat. Brain Res 579:321-326.

[74] Cooke, B.M., Tabibnia, G., Breedlove, S.M., 1999. A brain sexual dimorphism controlled by adult circulating androgens. Proc. Natl. Acad. Sci. U.S.A. 96, 7538-7540.

[75] Morris, J.A., Jordan, C.L., Breedlove, S.M., 2008 Sexual dimorphism in neuronal number of the

posterodorsal medial amygdala is independent of circulating androgens and regional volume in adult rats. J. Comp. Neurol. 506, 851-85.9

[76] Meaney, M.J., McEwen, B.S., 1986. Testosterone implants into the amygdala during the neonatal period masculinize the social play of juvenile female rats. Brain Res. 398, 324-328.

[77] Mizukami, S., Nishizuka, M., Arai, Y., 1983. Sexual difference in nuclear volume and its ontogeny in the rat amygdala. Exp. Neurol. 79, 569-575.

[78] Simerly, R.B., Chang, C., Muramatsu, M., Swanson, L.W., 1990. Distribution of androgen and estrogen receptor mRNA-containing cells in the rat brain: an in situ hybridization study. J. Comp. Neurol. 294, 76-95.

[79] Shughrue, P.J., Bushnell, C.D., Dorsa, D.M., 1992. Estrogen receptor messenger ribonucleic acid in female rat brain during the estrous cycle: a comparison with ovariectomized female and intact males. Endocrinology. 131, 381-388.

[80] Jakab, R.L., Horvath, T.L., Leranth, C., Harada, N., Naftolin, F., 1993. Aromatase immunoreactivity in the rat brain: gonadectomy-sensitive hypothalamic neurons and an unresponsive "limbic ring" of the lateral septum-bed nucleus-amygdala complex J. Steroid. Biochem. Mol. Biol. 44, 481-498.

[81] Roselli, C.E., Resko, J.A., 1997. Sex differences in androgen-regulated expression of cytochrome P450 aromatase in the rat brain. J. Steroid Biochem. Mol. Biol. 61, 7365-7466.

[82] Cooke, B.M., Breedlove, S.M., 2003. Cynthia L Jordan Both estrogen receptors and androgen receptors contribute to testosterone-induced changes in the morphology of the medial amygdala and sexual arousal in male rats. Horm. Behav. 43, 336-346.

[83] Morris, J.A., Jordan, C.L., Dugger, B.N., Breedlove, S.M., 2005. Partial demasculinization of several brain regions in adult male (XY) rats with a dysfunctional androgen receptor gene. J. Comp. Neurol. 487, 217-226.

[84] Cao, J., Heather B Patisaul, H.B., 2013. Sex-specific expression of estrogen receptors α and β and Kiss1 in the postnatal rat amygdala. J. Comp. Neurol. 521, 465-478.

[85] Chen, P.B., Hu, R.K., Wu, Y.E., Pan, L., Huang, S., Micevych, P.E., Hong, W., 2019.Sexually Dimorphic Control of Parenting Behavior by the Medial Amygdala. Cell. 176, 1206-1221.

[86] Hong, W., Dong-Wook Kim, D.W., David J Anderson, D.J., 2014. Antagonistic control of social versus repetitive self-grooming behaviors by separable amygdala neuronal subsets. Cell. 158, 1348-1361.

[87] Newman, S.W., 1999. The medial extended amygdala in male reproductive behavior. A node in the mammalian social behavior network. Ann. NY Acad. Sci. 877, 242-257.

[88] Gréco, B., Blasberg, M.E., Kosinski, E.C., Blaustein, J.D., 2003. Response of ERalpha-IR and ERbeta-IR cells in the forebrain of female rats to mating stimuli Horm. Behav. 43, 444-453.

[89] Kang, N., Baum, M.J., James A Cherry, J.A., 2009. A direct main olfactory bulb projection to the 'vomeronasal' amygdala in female mice selectively responds to volatile pheromones from males. Eur. J. Neurosci. 29, 624-634.

[90] Parvizi, N., Ellendorff, F., 1980. beta-Endorphin alters luteinizing hormone secretion via the amygdala but not the hypothalamus. Nature. 286, 812-813.

[91] Sanchez, M.A., Dominguez, R., 1995. Differential effects of unilateral

lesions in the medial amygdala on spontaneous and induced ovulation. Brain Res. Bull. 38, 313-317.

[92] Li, X.F., Hu, M.H., Hanley, B.P., Lin, Y.S., Poston, L., Lightman, S.L., O'Byrne K.T., 2015. The Posterodorsal Medial Amygdala Regulates the Timing of Puberty Onset in Female Rats. Endocrinology. 156, 3725-3736.

[93] Martel, K.L., Baum, M.J., 2009. A centrifugal pathway to the mouse accessory olfactory bulb from the medial amygdala conveys gender-specific volatile pheromonal signals. Eur. J. Neurosci. 29, 368-376.

Chapter 7

An Analysis of the Implication of Estrogens and Steroid Receptor Coactivators in the Genetic Basis of Gender Incongruence

Rosa Fernández, Karla Ramírez, Enrique Delgado-Zayas, Esther Gómez-Gil, Isabel Esteva, Antonio Guillamon and Eduardo Pásaro

Abstract

In mammals, sex differences in the adult brain are established very early in development, when the brain is still very immature. In the case of having inherited the *SRY* gene, during embryogenesis, testosterone secreted by the testes enters the brain and is converted to estradiol by the aromatase. Then the estradiol acts by binding to intracellular estrogen receptors (ERs) located predominantly in neurons, masculinizing specific brain regions. But ERs are also transcription factors that, when they are exposed to their ligand, dimerize and form complexes with coactivator proteins and corepressors, modifying the transcription of multiple target genes in a cascade effect and ultimately neuronal function. Given the intimate relationship between steroids and brain dimorphism, and steroid coactivators and gene transcription, in the present work, we further explore the implication of ERs α and β, and steroid coactivators NCoA-1, NCoA-2, NCoA-3, NCoA-4, NCoA-5 and p300-CREBBP, in the genesis of brain dimorphism. Based on our data, we believe that the coactivators NCOA-1, NCOA-2 and p300-CREBBP could be considered as candidate genes for GI.

Keywords: estrogens, gender incongruence, steroid coactivators

1. Introduction

1.1 Gender incongruence

The term *gender identity* refers to "a person's innermost concept of self as male, female, a blend of both or neither, how individuals perceive themselves and what they call themselves" [1, 2], while *sex* refers to the biological sex characteristics based on chromosomal, hormonal, physical, and anatomical characteristics.

Most people present an alignment of gender identity with natal sex (cisgender individuals), but in some cases (transgender individuals) gender identity differs (in varying degrees) from the sex assigned at birth. Thus, Gender Dysphoria (GD) in the Diagnostic and Statistical Manual of Mental Disorders DSM-5 [3] or Gender Incongruence (GI) in the International Classification of Diseases ICD-11 [4] are characterized by a marked incongruence between one's experienced gender and the sex assigned at birth.

2. The genetic and epigenetic basis of the gender incongruence

The origin of GI is complex and appears to be multifactorial. Current hypotheses point out that GI could be associated with a characteristic neurodevelopmental processes of the brain [5, 6], not concordant with gender, due to the influence of testosterone, converted into estradiol in the brain.

Traditionally, this process of brain masculinization *versus* feminization, has been exclusively analyzed from a hormonal perspective. But in the past two decades, it has been found that this point of view is incomplete, since other important factors such as epigenetics or genetics, for example, are not taken into account.

2.1 The genetic component

A genetic component should also be taken into account since different genes start to express before the formation of the testes [7, 8]. In fact, in mammals, sexual differentiation begins at the time of fertilization, through a different chromosomal complement in males and females, and will be driven by the *SRY* gene, which will guide the undifferentiated gonad towards the formation of the testes. Then, the testosterone will masculinize specific regions of the brain, either directly, or indirectly, through the action of the aromatase [9, 10].

Most studies about the genetic basis of GI analyzed the implication of some DNA polymorphisms related to ERs, α and β, the AR, the aromatase CYP19A1 or the CYP17A1 [11–20] as well as the interaction effects (epistasis) among them [15, 21]. A summary of the principal studies about the genetic component of GI is shown in **Table 1**. This gene selection is based on the hypothesis that a small variation in the DNA sequence of these genes would imply a high variability in the sensitivity of the hormonal receptors to their ligands.

Henningsson et al. [11] were the first group to analyze three repeat polymorphisms, located in the estrogen receptor beta, the androgen receptor, and the aromatase genes in a trans female population. They found a relationship between the number of repetitions and gender incongruence. They found longer estrogen receptor and androgen receptor polymorphisms in the trans female population. Later, Hare et al. [12] replicated Henningsson's study in a bigger population, finding longer androgen receptor polymorphisms. However, when Ujike et al., [13] analyzed the same polymorphisms in a Japanese population, they did not find any statistical difference. These and others polymorphisms were analyzed in a Spanish population by our group. Our results confirmed the involvement of both estrogen receptors (alpha and beta) in gender incongruence. Part of this data was confirmed by Foreman et al. [15].

2.2 The epigenetic component

An epigenetic component may also be involved since there is evidence that some environmental factors play a role in the sexual differentiation of the brain. For example, in mice, the sex difference in maternal anogenital licking of male compared with female pups produces a different methylation of the estrogen receptor α promoter in the preoptic area [22]. And in humans, certain environmental factors, such as a short crossover hormonal treatment (only 6 months), can modify the methylation profile of the estrogen receptor α promoter in a trans population [23, 24].

Investigations	Genes	Populations
Henningsson et al. [11]	ERβ, AR, CYP19A1	29 transwomen
Hare et al. [12]	ERβ, AR, CYP19A1	112 transwomen
Ujikce et al. [13]	ERβ, AR, CYP19A1	168 transmen 74 transwomen
Fernández et al. [14, 16]	ERβ, AR, CYP19A1	273 transmen 442 transwomen
Bentz et al. [19]	CYP17A1	49 transmen 104 transwomen
Fernández et al. [20] (2016)	CYP17A1	223 transmen 317 transwomen
Cortés Cortés et al. [17]	ERα: (TA)n-rs3138774, PvuII-rs2234693, XbaI-rs9340799	183 transmen 184 transwomen
Fernández et al. [21]	ERα, ERβ, AR, CYP19A	425 transmen 549 transwomen
Foreman et al. [15]	AR, ERα, ERβ, SRD5A2, STS, SULT2A1, PGR, COMT, CYP17, SRD5A2	380 transwomen
Fernández et al. [18]	ERα: rs9478245, rs3138774 rs2234693, rs9340799	226 transmen 273 transwomen
Aranda et al. [24]	Epigenetics: ERα, ERβ, AR	12 transmen 6 transwomen
Fernández et al. [23]	Epigenetics: ERα promoter	10 transmen 10 transwomen

Table 1.
Mean investigations about the genetic basis of gender incongruence.

3. Estrogens, androgens and their receptors and coactivators

3.1 Estrogens

Estradiol (E2) exerts a wide variety of effects on growth, development, the function of reproductive systems and regulation in the central nervous system [25, 26]. The mechanism of action of the two ER isoforms α and β consists of binding with the E2 ligand to obtain the receptor's dimerization (αα, αβ or ββ), originating the necessary conformational changes in the ligand binding domain (LBD) [27] and binding with high affinity to specific DNA sequences called estrogen response elements (EREs) [27] in the genes that are regulated by E2 (**Figure 1**). This conformational change in the LBD allows coactivators and other co-regulating proteins to be recruited. We must point out that this step is critical for the transcriptional regulation of genes induced by E2 [28].

Furthermore, estrogens are produced in many regions of the brain including the cortex, the hippocampus, the cerebellum, the hypothalamus and the amygdala, among others [29]. The actions of estrogens in the developing brain are generally permanent and range from the establishment of sexual differences to generalized trophic and neuroprotective effects [30]. In addition, estrogens are an important regulator of brain growth and differentiation, and ERs α and β are found in both the developing [31] and the adult human brain [32].

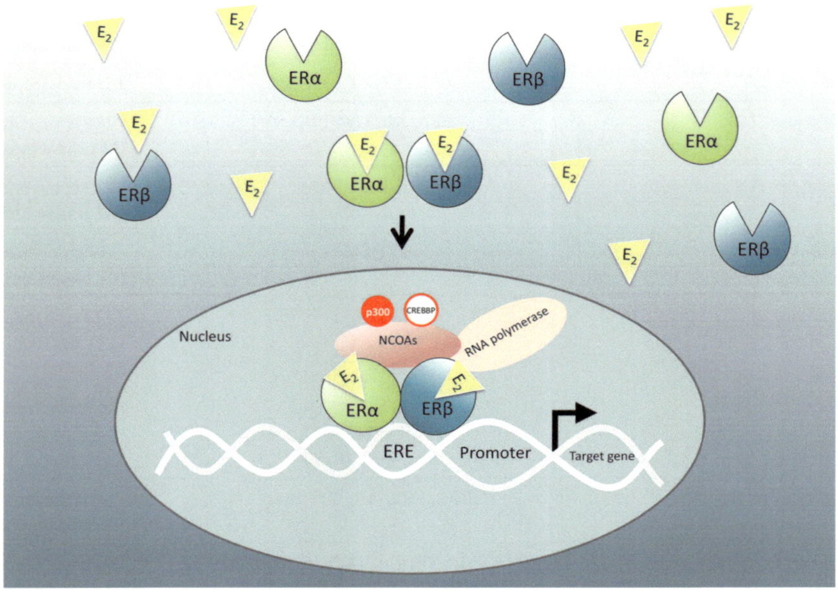

Figure 1.
Molecular mechanisms of action of ERs α and β. hormone 17β-estradiol (E2) binds to the nuclear receptor (ERα or ERβ), and after dimerization and translocation to the nucleus, the nuclear receptor complex binds to a specific sequence of DNA known as an estrogen response element (ERE). The nuclear receptor complex in turn recruits the coactivators NCOAs, p300 and the CREBBP that activate the transcription of target genes.

3.2 Estrogen and androgen receptors are transcription factors

We must point out that the packaging of DNA into chromatin causes a general repression of gene activity, and transcription factors function to relieve this chromatin-mediated repression [33].Thereby, once attached to their ligands, the receptors dimerize, enter the nucleus, and interact with the promoter regions of the target genes, modulating the expression of multiple genes in collaboration with some steroid coactivators (**Figure 1**). In the case of the AR, its ligand is androgen [34] while for the ERs, it is estrogen, 17β-Estradiol (E2) in particular [26].

3.3 Steroid receptor coactivators

Proteins called SRCs (Steroid Receptor Coactivators) serve as primary coactivators that interact with the complex formed by E2 and the hormonal receptor. Additionally, SRCs recruit multiple secondary coactivators such as p300 and the CREB-binding protein (also known as CREBBP) [35]. Both SRCs and p300 are the first coactivators that are coupled to the E2-ER complex [36] to activate the transcriptional process of the genes that are E2 targets (**Figure 1**).

Coactivators are proteins that influence the ability of the transcription factors to activate or inhibit expression of multiple genes in a cascade mode [37]. Given the intimate relationship between steroids and brain dimorphism, and coactivators and gene transcription, and since ERs α-β and the AR are hormonal receptors that act as transcription factors, it was clear that we should hypothesize the implication of DNA coactivators in the process of GI.

4. The role of E2-coactivators in the genetic basis of gender incongruence

To our knowledge, no studies have been published about the role of steroid receptor coactivators in the genetic basis of GI. Nevertheless, given the importance of estrogens in GI, and the critical role of coactivators in the transcriptional gene regulation induced by E2, our team deemed it interesting to analyze 247 single nucleotide polymorphisms (SNPs) located at the coactivators NCoA-1(or SRC-1), NCoA-2 (or SRC-2), NCoA-3 (or SRC-3), NCoA-4, NCoA-5 and p300-CREBBP, in a transgender *versus* a cisgender population, because variation at the DNA level at steroid receptor coactivators could affect the sensitivity of the E2-ER complex, and consequently could modify the transcription of the genes regulated by E2. Some of these data are being published, and the results of the whole study are presented in this chapter.

4.1 The characteristics of the study

Genomic DNA was extracted from 94 Spanish transgender individuals (47 transmen and 47 transwomen) *versus* 94 Spanish cis gender individuals (44 cismen and 50 ciswomen). The transgender population was diagnosed and recruited through the Gender Unit of the Clínic Hospital of Barcelona (Spain) and the cisgender population was selected from a country census (Pizarra) matching by geographic origin and race.

We analyzed 247 polymorphisms distributed in the coactivators NCOA-1 (63 SNPs), NCOA-2 (64 SNPs), NCOA-3 (30 SNPs), NCOA-4 (4 SNPs), NCOA-5 (8 SNPs), p300 (9 SNPs) and CREBBP (69 SNPs) (**Table 2**), in a population of 94 Spanish transgender individuals *versus* 94 Spanish cisgender individuals, with the same geographic origin, race and biological sex. All the polymorphisms were in Hardy–Weinberg equilibrium.

4.2 The findings

4.2.1 Similar prevalence rates for the analyzed polymorphisms and comparison with the global and European 1000 genomes

As expected, the prevalence rates for all analyzed polymorphisms in our population were similar to those found in the Global 1000 genomes and the European 1000 genomes http://www.1000genomes.org (**Table 3**).

4.2.2 Eleven polymorphism showed differences in the distribution of the allele and genotype frequencies

When we compared the distribution of the allele and genotype frequencies, we found significant differences in 11 polymorphisms, that correspond to 4.45% of the total analyzed: three polymorphisms located in NCOA-1, five in NCOA-2, two in p300 and one in CREBBP (**Tables 2** and **3**). The description of the significant association analyses with GI in different models of inheritance is in **Table 4**.

P1 polymorphism: The genotype T/T was overrepresented in the cis population ($P < 0.035$ for dominant model) while the genotypes T/C-C/C were more frequent in the trans population (OR = 2.12; $P < 0.038$). The genotype distribution was also significant for the log-additive model (OR = 2.15; $P < 0.027$).

Gene	Chromosome	Function	Analyzed SNPs	SNPs with significant differences
NCOA-1	2	The protein encoded by this gene acts as a transcriptional coactivator for steroid and nuclear hormone receptors.	63	3
NCOA-2	8	The encoded protein acts as an intermediary factor for the ligand-dependent activity of nuclear receptors, which regulate their target genes upon binding of cognate response elements.	64	5
NCOA-3	20	The protein encoded by this gene is a nuclear receptor coactivator that interacts with nuclear hormone receptors to enhance their transcriptional activator functions.	30	0
NCOA-4	10	This gene encodes an androgen receptor coactivator.	4	0
NCOA-5	20	This gene encodes a coregulator for the α and β estrogen receptors.	8	0
p300	22	This gene encodes a transcriptional coactivator protein.	9	2
CREBBP	16	This gene is ubiquitously expressed and is involved in the transcriptional coactivation factors.	69	1
		TOTAL	**247**	**11**
		%	**100**	**4.45**

Table 2.
Description of the analyzed polymorphisms.

Gene	Polymorphism	Alias	DNA variation	Our study frequency	Global 1000 genomes frequency	European 1000 genomes frequency
NCOA-1	rs10495747	P1	T/C	C = 0.11	C = 0.1330	C = 0.1153
	rs2584940	P2	T/G	G = 0.38	G = 0.4605	G = 0.4125
	rs6756785	P3	A/G	G = 0.32	G = 0.2115	G = 0.2883
NCOA-2	rs76968380	P4	G/A	A = 0.06	A = 0.1138	A = 0.0646
	rs34406737	P5	G/A	A = 0.15	A = 0.1300	A = 0.1262
	rs1963250	P6	G/T	T = 0.57	T = 0.5691	T = 0.5368
	rs10755950	P7	G/A	A = 0.42	A = 0.5655	A = 0.4483
	rs56055423	P8	A/G	G = 0.05	G = 0.0132	G = 0.0457
p300	rs133084	P9	T/C	C = 0.5956	C = 0.5447	C = 0.59
	rs11806	P10	A/G	G = 0.3894	G = 0.3499	G = 0.42
CREBBP	rs2191416	P11	G/A	A = 0.2660	A = 0.2555	A = 0.26

Table 3.
Description of the polymorphisms with significant differences.

P2 polymorphism: The genotype T/T was overrepresented in the cis population ($P < 0.044$), while the genotypes T/G (OR = 1.97; $P < 0.035$) and G/G (OR = 2.65; $P < 0.045$) were overrepresented in the trans population (codominant model). The genotype distribution for P2 was also significant for the dominant and log-additive models.

P3 polymorphism: The genotype A/A was overrepresented in the cis population ($P < 0.0079$ for the dominant model), while the genotypes A/G-G/G were overrepresented in the trans population (OR = 2.20; $P < 0.009$). The genotype distribution for P3 was significant for the codominant, dominant, overdominant and log-additive models.

P4 polymorphism: The P4 polymorphism was only significant for the log-additive model. The genotype G/G was overrepresented in the cis population, while the genotypes G/A and A/A were overrepresented in the trans population (OR = 2.57; $P < 0.034$ for the log-additive model).

P5 polymorphism: This polymorphism was significant for the codominant, the recessive, and the overdominant models. The G/G and the A/A genotypes were overrepresented in the trans population ($P < 0.0029$; codominant model)) while the G/A was overrepresented in the cis population (OR = 0.48; $P < 0.036$).

P6 polymorphism: The T/T genotype was overrepresented in the trans population while the T/G and G/G were overrepresented in the cis population (OR = 0.42; $P < 0.008$ for the dominant model). The genotype distribution was significant for the codominant, dominant and log-additive models.

P7 polymorphism: This polymorphism was only significant for the recessive model. The A/A genotype was overrepresented in the trans population (OR = 2.44; $P < 0.026$, recessive model).

P8 polymorphism: The genotype A/A was overrepresented in the cis population ($P < 0.0068$ dominant model) while the genotype A/G was overrepresented in the trans population (OR = 4.49; $P < 0.024$, codominant model). This polymorphism showed significant differences for the codominant, dominant, overdominant, and log-additive models. Only the recessive model did not show significant results.

P9 polymorphism: The C/C genotype was overrepresented in the trans population, while the T/C and T/T were overrepresented in the cis population (OR = 0.50; $P < 0.025$, dominant model).

P10 polymorphism: This polymorphism was only significant for the log-additive model. The G/G genotype was overrepresented in the trans population (OR = 2.69; $P < 0.030$, codominant model).

P11 polymorphism: The A/A polymorphism was overrepresented in the trans population (OR = 4.82; $P < 0.048$, recessive model), while G/G-A/G were more frequent in the cis population ($P < 0.025$).

4.2.3 The three polymorphisms (P2, P9 and P10) showed significant differences in the interaction analysis with the covariate "sex"

Furthermore, polymorphisms P2, P9 and P10 showed significant differences in the interaction analysis with covariate "sex". For the P2 polymorphism, the genotype T/G was more frequent in the trans population assigned as females at birth than in the cis female population (OR = 2.76; $P < 0.029$) while the genotype G/G was more frequent in the trans population assigned as males than in the cis male population (OR = 8.0; $P < 0.016$).

While for the P9 polymorphism, the genotype T/T was more frequent in the cis female population than in the trans population assigned as females at birth (OR = 0.34; $P < 0.014$). And finally, the genotypes A/G-G/G for the P10 polymorphism were more frequent in the trans population assigned as females at birth than in the cis female population (OR = 2.68; $P < 0.031$).

Model	Genotype	Cis (%)	Trans (%)	OR	*P*-value
P1 polymorphism (rs10495747)					
Codominant	T/T	79 (84%)	67 (71.3%)	1.00	0.068
	T/C	15 (16%)	26 (27.7%)	2.04 (1.00–4.17)	**0.05***
	C/C	0 (0%)	1 (1.1%)	NA (0.00-NA)	—
Dominant	T/T	79 (84%)	67 (71.3%)	1.00	**0.035***
	T/C-C/C	15 (16%)	27 (28.7%)	2.12 (1.04–4.32)	**0.038***
Recessive	T/T–T/C	94 (100%)	93 (98.9%)	1.00	0.24
	C/C	0 (0%)	1 (1.1%)	NA (0.00-NA)	—
Overdominant	T/T-C/C	79 (84%)	68 (72.3%)	1.00	0.051
	T/C	15 (16%)	26 (27.7%)	2.01 (0.99–4.11)	0,054
Log-additive	—	—	—	2.15 (1.07–4.29)	**0.027***
P2 polymorphism (rs2584940)					
Codominant	T/T	43 (45.7%)	27 (28.7%)	1.00	**0.044***
	T/G	42 (44.7%)	52 (55.3%)	1.97 (1.05–3.70)	**0.035***
	G/G	9 (9.6%)	15 (16%)	2.65 (1.02–6.91)	**0.045***
Dominant	T/T	43 (45.7%)	27 (28.7%)	1.00	**0.015***
	T/G-G/G	51 (54.3%)	67 (71.3%)	2.09 (1.14–3.83)	**0.017***
Recessive	T/T–T/G	85 (90.4%)	79 (84%)	1.00	0.19
	G/G	9 (9.6%)	15 (16%)	1.79 (0.74–4.33)	0.198
Overdominant	T/T-G/G	52 (55.3%)	42 (44.7%)	1.00	0.14
	T/G	42 (44.7%)	52 (55.3%)	1.53 (0.86–2.72)	0.148
Log-additive	—	—	—	1.72 (1.10–2.69)	**0.015***
P3 polymorphism (rs6756785)					
Codominant	A/A	50 (53.2%)	32 (34%)	1.00	**0.029***
	A/G	38 (40.4%)	54 (57.5%)	2.22 (1.21–4.08)	**0.010***
	G/G	6 (6.4%)	8 (8.5%)	2.08 (0.66–6.56)	0.213
Dominant	A/A	50 (53.2%)	32 (34%)	1.00	**0.0079***
	A/G-G/G	44 (46.8%)	62 (66%)	2.20 (1.22–3.97)	**0.009***
Recessive	A/A-A/G	88 (93.6%)	86 (91.5%)	1.00	0.58
	G/G	6 (6.4%)	8 (8.5%)	1.36 (0.45–4.10)	0.598
Overdominant	A/A-G/G	56 (59.6%)	40 (42.5%)	1.00	**0.019***
	A/G	38 (40.4%)	54 (57.5%)	1.99 (1.11–3.55)	**0.020***
Log-additive	—	—	—	1.77 (1.10–2.87)	**0.017***
P4 polymorphism (rs76968380)					
Codominant	G/G	88 (93.6%)	80 (85.1%)	1.00	0.075
	G/A	6 (6.4%)	12 (12.8%)	2.20 (0.79–6.14)	0.132
	A/A	0 (0%)	2 (2.1%)	NA (0.00-NA)	—
Dominant	G/G	88 (93.6%)	80 (85.1%)	1.00	0.055
	G/A-A/A	6 (6.4%)	14 (14.9%)	2.57 (0.94–7.00)	0.065

Model	Genotype	Cis (%)	Trans (%)	OR	*P*-value
Recessive	G/G-G/A	94 (100%)	92 (97.9%)	1.00	0.095
	A/A	0 (0%)	2 (2.1%)	NA (0.00-NA)	—
Overdominant	G/G-A/A	88 (93.6%)	82 (87.2%)	1.00	0.13
	G/A	6 (6.4%)	12 (12.8%)	2.15 (0.77–5.98)	0.144
Log-additive	—	—	—	2.57 (1.01–6.55)	**0.034***
P5 polymorphism (rs34406737)					
Codominant	G/G	63 (67%)	72 (76.6%)	1.00	**0.0029***
	G/A	31 (33%)	17 (18.1%)	0.48 (0.24–0.95)	**0.036***
	A/A	0 (0%)	5 (5.3%)	NA (0.00-NA)	—
Dominant	G/G	63 (67%)	72 (76.6%)	1.00	0.14
	G/A-A/A	31 (33%)	22 (23.4%)	0.62 (0.33–1.18)	0.142
Recessive	G/G-G/A	94 (100%)	89 (94.7%)	1.00	**0.0078***
	A/A	0 (0%)	5 (5.3%)	NA (0.00-NA)	—
Overdominant	G/G-A/A	63 (67%)	77 (81.9%)	1.00	**0.018***
	G/A	31 (33%)	17 (18.1%)	0.45 (0.23–0.88)	**0.020***
Log-additive	—	—	—	0.85 (0.49–1.49)	0.57
P6 polymorphism (rs1963250)					
Codominant	T/T	20 (21.3%)	37 (39.4%)	1.00	**0.015***
	T/G	54 (57.5%)	46 (48.9%)	0.46 (0.24–0.90)	**0.021***
	G/G	20 (21.3%)	11 (11.7%)	0.30 (0.12–0.74)	**0.009***
Dominant	T/T	20 (21.3%)	37 (39.4%)	1.00	**0.0067***
	T/G-G/G	74 (78.7%)	57 (60.6%)	0.42 (0.22–0.79)	**0.008***
Recessive	T/T–T/G	74 (78.7%)	83 (88.3%)	1.00	0.075
	G/G	20 (21.3%)	11 (11.7%)	0.49 (0.22–1.09)	0.080
Overdominant	T/T-G/G	40 (42.5%)	48 (51.1%)	1.00	0.24
	T/G	54 (57.5%)	46 (48.9%)	0.71 (0.40–1.26)	0.245
Log-additive	—	—	—	0.53 (0.34–0.83)	**0.0043***
P7 polymorphism (rs10755950)					
Codominant	G/G	33 (35.1%)	31 (33%)	1.00	0.064
	A/G	50 (53.2%)	40 (42.5%)	0.85 (0.45–1.62)	0.632
	A/A	11 (11.7%)	23 (24.5%)	2.23 (0.93–5.31)	0.071
Dominant	G/G	33 (35.1%)	31 (33%)	1.00	0.76
	A/G-A/A	61 (64.9%)	63 (67%)	1.10 (0.60–2.01)	0.770
Recessive	G/G-A/G	83 (88.3%)	71 (75.5%)	1.00	**0.022***
	A/A	11 (11.7%)	23 (24.5%)	2.44 (1.11–5.36)	**0.026***
Overdominant	G/G-A/A	44 (46.8%)	54 (57.5%)	1.00	0.14
	A/G	50 (53.2%)	40 (42.5%)	0.65 (0.37–1.16)	0.14
Log-additive	—	—	—	1.35 (0.90–2.04)	0.15

Model	Genotype	Cis (%)	Trans (%)	OR	*P*-value
P8 polymorphism (rs56055423)					
Codominant	A/A	91 (96.8%)	81 (86.2%)	1.00	**0.021***
	A/G	3 (3.2%)	12 (12.8%)	4.49 (1.22–16.49)	**0.024***
	G/G	0 (0%)	1 (1.1%)	NA (0.00-NA)	—
Dominant	A/A	91 (96.8%)	81 (86.2%)	1.00	**0.0068***
	A/G-G/G	3 (3.2%)	13 (13.8%)	4.87 (1.34–17.69)	**0.016***
Recessive	A/A-A/G	94 (100%)	93 (98.9%)	1.00	0.24
	G/G	0 (0%)	1 (1.1%)	NA (0.00-NA)	—
Overdominant	A/A-G/G	91 (96.8%)	82 (87.2%)	1.00	**0.012***
	A/G	3 (3.2%)	12 (12.8%)	4.44 (1.21–16.29)	**0.024***
Log-additive	—	—	—	4.69 (1.32–16.63)	**0.0057***
P9 polymorphism (rs133084)					
Codominant	C/C	27 (28.7%)	42 (44.7%)	1.00	0.056
	T/C	46 (48.9%)	39 (41.5%)	0.55 (0.29–1.04)	0.066
	T/T	21 (22.3%)	13 (13.8%)	0.40 (0.17–0.93)	**0.034***
Dominant	C/C	27 (28.7%)	42 (44.7%)	1.00	**0.023***
	T/C-T/T	67 (71.3%)	52 (55.3%)	0.50 (0.27–0.91)	**0.025***
Recessive	C/C-T/C	73 (77.7%)	81 (86.2%)	1.00	0.13
	T/T	21 (22.3%)	13 (13.8%)	0.56 (0.26–1.19)	0.135
Overdominant	C/C-T/T	48 (51.1%)	55 (58.5%)	1.00	0.3
	T/C	46 (48.9%)	39 (41.5%)	0.74 (0.42–1.32)	0.307
Log-additive	—	—	—	0.61 (0.41–0.93)	**0.019***
P10 polymorphism (rs11806)					
Codominant	A/A	37 (39.8%)	25 (26.6%)	1.00	0.076
	A/G	45 (48.4%)	49 (52.1%)	1.61 (0.84–3.08)	0.151
	G/G	11 (11.8%)	20 (21.3%)	2.69 (1.10–6.58)	**0.030***
Dominant	A/A	37 (39.8%)	25 (26.6%)	1.00	0.055
	A/G-G/G	56 (60.2%)	69 (73.4%)	1.82 (0.98–3.38)	0.058
Recessive	A/A-A/G	82 (88.2%)	74 (78.7%)	1.00	0.08
	G/G	11 (11.8%)	20 (21.3%)	2.01 (0.91–4.48)	0.086
Overdominant	A/A-G/G	48 (51.6%)	45 (47.9%)	1.00	0.61
	A/G	45 (48.4%)	49 (52.1%)	1.16 (0.65–2.06)	0.627
Log-additive	—	—	—	1.63 (1.06–2.52)	**0.023***
P11 polymorphism (rs2191416)					
Codominant	G/G	53 (57%)	47 (50%)	1.00	0.075
	A/G	38 (40.9%)	38 (40.4%)	1.13 (0.62–2.05)	0.702
	A/A	2 (2.1%)	9 (9.6%)	5.07 (1.04–24.67)	**0.044***
Dominant	G/G	53 (57%)	47 (50%)	1.00	0.34
	A/G-A/A	40 (43%)	47 (50%)	1.32 (0.74–2.36)	0.354
Recessive	G/G-A/G	91 (97.8%)	85 (90.4%)	1.00	**0.025***
	A/A	2 (2.1%)	9 (9.6%)	4.82 (1.01–22.93)	**0.048***

Model	Genotype	Cis (%)	Trans (%)	OR	*P*-value
Overdominant	G/G-A/A	55 (59.1%)	56 (59.6%)	1.00	0.95
	A/G	38 (40.9%)	38 (40.4%)	0.98 (0.55–1.76)	0.951
Log-additive	—	—	—	1.49 (0.92–2.41)	0.1

Table 4.
Polymorphism association analysis with gender incongruence, in different models of inheritance (Codominant, Dominant, Recessive, Overdominant and Log-additive) (n = 188, crude analysis).

4.2.4 The haplotype analysis of the coactivators NCOA-1, NCOA-2 and p300, and comparison between cis and trans population

The simultaneous analysis of multiple loci (haplotypes) was carried out in those coactivators with two or more polymorphisms with statistical significance (NCOA-1, NCOA-2 and p300) using logistic regression models.

4.2.4.1 Polymorphisms in NCOA-1

For the three polymorphisms located in NCOA-1 (**Table 5**), the T allele for P1 was linked to the T allele for P2, and to the A allele for P3 (haplotype 1: T–T-A) with a total frequency of 0.45. This haplotype was more frequent in the cis than in the trans population. The haplotype 5: C-G-A was overrepresented in the trans population and showed statistical significance (OR = 2.62; $P < 0.05$). The P global haplotype association was $P < 0.009$.

4.2.4.2 Polymorphisms in NCOA-2

For the five polymorphisms located in NCOA-2 (**Table 6**), the significant haplotypes were the haplotype 2: (G-G-T-A-A) (OR = 2.49; $P < 0.02$) and the haplotype 8: (G-G-T-A-G) (OR = 12.86; $P < 0.028$), with a P global haplotype association $P < 0.005$. Both polymorphisms were overrepresented in the trans population.

4.2.4.3 Polymorphisms in p300

For the two polymorphisms located in p300 (**Table 7**), the significant haplotype was haplotype 2 (T-A) (OR = 0.57; $P < 0.018$) with a P global haplotype association $P < 0.033$. This haplotype was more frequent in the cis than in the trans population, and it was only significant in the population with a female natal sex (biological sex) (OR = 0.43; $P < 0.013$) (**Table 8**).

4.2.4.4 Summary of findings

In summary, when we analyzed the allele and genotype frequencies, we found significant differences in 11 polymorphisms located in NCOA-1, NCOA-2, p300 and CREBBP. Being the NCOA-2 and p300 the coactivators with the highest percentages of polymorphisms with significant differences (5/64 and 2/9 respectively). Furthermore, only P2 (located at NCOA-1), P9 (located at p300) and P10 (located at p300) showed a different distribution of the genotypes in males and females, that is, they showed significant differences in the interaction analysis with covariate "sex".

Regarding the haplotype analysis, there were four polymorphisms with significant differences: the haplotype 5 (C-G-A) in NCOA-1, the haplotype 2

Haplotype frequencies estimation and haplotype association with GI (n = 188, adjusted by sex)									
Haplotypes	**P1**	**P2**	**P3**	**Total**	**Cis population**	**Trans population**	**Cumulative frequency**	**OR (95% CI)**	***P*-value**
1	T	T	A	0.4501	0.5201	0.377	0.4501	1.00	—
2	T	T	G	0.1495	0.134	0.1699	0.5996	2.25 (0.99–5.13)	0.054
3	T	G	G	0.147	0.1319	0.1601	0.7466	1.73 (0.81–3.71)	0.16
4	T	G	A	0.139	0.1341	0.144	0.8856	1.80 (0.81–3.97)	0.15
5	C	G	A	0.069	0.0531	0.0897	0.9546	2.62 (1.00–6.83)	**0.05***
6	C	T	A	0.0228	0.0267	0.0169	0.9774	1.39 (0.23–8.34)	0.72
7	C	G	G	0.0226	0	0.0423	1	379142884.10 (379142883.16–379142885.04)	**<0.0001***

**Global haplotype association* P*-value: 0.009.*

Table 5.
Haplotype analysis for polymorphisms located in NCOA-1 (P1, P2 and P3 polymorphisms).

Haplotype frequencies estimation and haplotype association with GI (n = 188, adjusted by sex)											
Haplotypes	**P4**	**P5**	**P6**	**P7**	**P8**	**Total**	**Cis population**	**Trans population**	**Cumulative frequency**	**OR (95% CI)**	**P-value**
1	G	G	G	G	A	0.2546	0.3239	0.1963	0.2546	1.00	—
2	G	G	T	A	A	0.2206	0.2142	0.236	0.4752	2.49 (1.16–5.34)	**0.02***
3	G	G	T	G	A	0.2022	0.1721	0.2303	0.6773	2.00 (0.93–4.31)	0.079
4	G	G	G	A	A	0.0891	0.0861	0.0793	0.7664	1.05 (0.38–2.88)	0.92
5	G	A	G	G	A	0.0474	0.0656	0.0235	0.8138	0.55 (0.11–2.89)	0.48
6	G	A	T	A	A	0.0419	0.0474	0.0423	0.8557	1.11 (0.24–5.24)	0.89
7	G	A	T	G	A	0.041	0.0393	0.0426	0.8967	3.00 (0.10–86.09)	0.52
8	G	G	T	A	G	0.0217	0	0.036	0.9184	12.86 (1.34–123.38)	**0.028***
9	A	G	T	G	A	0.0173	0.0085	0.0228	0.9357	5.62 (0.56–56.71)	0.15
10	A	G	G	G	A	0.0165	0.0077	0.0205	0.9522	3.53 (0.40–31.50)	0.26
11	G	A	T	A	G	0.0138	0.0028	0.0189	0.9659	2.68 (0.27–26.20)	0.4
12	A	G	T	A	A	0.0108	0.0158	0.0093	0.9767	0.00 (-Inf - Inf)	1
rare	*	*	*	*	*				1	268876742466656413941852925381944582495847650337136368439787 52.00 (268876742466228467993671970371208066030767913715443365692047 36.00–268876742467084359890033880392681098960927386958829371187527 68.00)	**<0.0001***

Global haplotype association P-value: 0.005.

Table 6.
Haplotype analysis for polymorphisms located in NCOA-2 (P4, P5, P6, P7 and P8 polymorphisms).

Haplotype frequencies estimation and Haplotype association with GI (n = 188, adjusted by sex)								
Haplotypes	**P9**	**P10**	**Total**	**Cis population**	**Trans population**	**Cumulative frequency**	**OR (95% CI)**	***P*-value**
1	C	G	0.4103	0.3468	0.4734	0.4103	1.00	—
2	T	A	0.4004	0.4549	0.3457	0.8107	0.57 (0.36–0.90)	**0.018***
3	C	A	0.1828	0.1851	0.1809	0.9935	0.69 (0.38–1.27)	0.24
4	T	G	0.0065	0.0132	0	1	0.00 (-Inf - Inf)	1

Global haplotype association P-value: 0.033.

Table 7.
Haplotype analysis for polymorphisms located in p300 (P9 and P10 polymorphisms).

Haplotype and sex cross-classification interaction table (n = 188, crude analysis)					
		Females		**Males**	
Haplotype	**Frequency**	**OR (95% CI)**	***P*-value**	**OR (95% CI)**	***P*-value**
1	0.4102	1.00	—	0.63 (0.19–2.07)	0.457
2	0.4003	0.43 (0.22–0.83)	**0.013***	0.49 (0.19–1.27)	0.141
3	0.1829	0.60 (0.26–1.40)	0.237	0.52 (0.18–1.52)	0.232
Rare	0.0066	0.00 (0.00 - Inf)	—	0.00 (-Inf - Inf)	—
Haplotypes within sex (n = 188, crude analysis)					
		Females		**Males**	
Haplotype	**Frequency**	**OR (95% CI)**	***P*-value**	**OR (95% CI)**	***P*-value**
1	0.4102	1.00	—	1.00	—
2	0.4003	0.43 (0.22–0.83)	**0.013***	0.77 (0.40–1.49)	0.444
3	0.1829	0.60 (0.26–1.40)	0.237	0.82 (0.35–1.96)	0.665
Rare	0.0066	0.00 (0.00 - Inf)	—	0.00 (0.00 - Inf)	—
Sex within haplotypes (n = 188, crude analysis)					
		Females	**Males**		
Haplotype	**Frequency**	**OR (95% CI)**	**OR (95% CI)**	***P*-value**	
1	0.4102	1.00	0.63 (0.19–2.07)	0.457	
2	0.4003	1.00	1.12 (0.55–2.30)	0.769	
3	0.1829	1.00	0.87 (0.32–2.34)	0.796	
Rare	0.0066	1.00	Inf		

Table 8.
Haplotype interaction analysis with covariate sex for polymorphisms located in p300 (P9 and P10 polymorphisms). Haplotype frequency, Odds ratio (OR) and P-value in female and male populations.

(G-G-T-A-A) in NCOA-2, the haplotype 8 (G-G-T-A-G) also in NCOA-2, and the haplotype 2 (T-A) in p300. These NCOA-1 and NCOA-2 significant haplotypes were more frequent in the trans population (OR = 2.62, OR = 2.49 and OR = 12.86, respectively) while the haplotype 2 (T-A) in p300 was more frequent in the cis population (OR = 0.57). The NCOA-2 haplotype 8 (OR = 12.86; $P < 0.028$) had a strikingly much higher value than the others. That is due to the fact that this haplotype only occurred in the trans population.

4.3 Concordance of our findings with the literature about receptor coactivators

To our knowledge, no studies have been published about the role of steroid receptor coactivators in the genetic basis of GI. Our data are in concordance with a recent work that showed that the nuclear receptor coactivators, NCOA-1, NCOA-2 and p300, are essential for efficient ER transcriptional activity in the brain [33, 38]. Furthermore, NCOA-1 and NCOA-2 are distributed in several specific areas of the brain in different proportions, such as the hypothalamus and the hippocampus, showing at the same time, difference in the coupling with the ERs [38, 39]. These differential interactions between NCOA-1 and NCOA-2 with the ER subtypes α and β suggest that these brain regions have distinct expression pattern of co-regulators, and understanding how nuclear receptor coactivators function with various steroid receptors is critical to understanding how hormones act in different brain regions.

Moreover, our results are also in concordance with the study of the functional significance of the nuclear receptor coactivator NCOA-1 in the developing brain [40]. The authors, Auger et al., investigated the consequence of reducing NCOA-1 protein during sexual differentiation of the brain, and reported that reducing this protein interferes with the defeminizing actions of estrogen in neonatal rat brains. Their data indicated that NCOA-1 expression is critically involved in the hormone-dependent development of normal male reproductive behavior and brain morphology. Thus, our data are in agreement with the results of Auger et al., [40] since the polymorphic analysis of this coactivator showed significant differences when allelic and genotypic frequencies and haplotypes analyses were carried out.

Our data are also in concordance with other studies about the critical role of p300 and CREBBP in ERα transcription. p300 and CREBBP are two of multiple secondary coactivators recruited by NCOA1, NCOA2 or NCOA3 to form a receptor-coactivator complex that can promote chromatin remodeling and facilitate transcriptional activation [35]. In our work, we found statistical significances in p300, CREBBP, NCOA1 and NCOA2, but not in NCOA3.

Transcription by RNA polymerase II requires the coordinated action of multiple factors such as DNA-binding factors, coactivators, chromatin remodeling, with the basal transcriptional machinery. Futhermore, p300 and CREBBP, do not bind DNA on their own, but they play an essential role in the transcription process mediated by E2 [33, 41]. Thus, ERα functions cooperatively with p300 and CREBBP to increase transcription [42]. Yi et al. [35] demonstrated the quaternary structure of an active complex of DNA-bound ERα, steroid receptor coactivator, and p300 as secondary coactivator. The structural model suggests that the ER binds the ERE-DNA as a dimer and then recruits two NCOAs; these two coactivators, in turn, secure one molecule of p300 to the complex through multiple contacts.

It is very important to maintain the nucleotide sequence of the genes encoding the coactivators in order to maintain the interactions of the ER-E2 -NCOA -p300-CREBBP complex and thus perform the genomic function of estrogens. Therefore, our data are in concordance because finding significant polymorphisms in the sample analyzed may result in ineffective or low effective interactions affecting the E2 target genes involved in brain dimorphism.

In our work, we found 2/9 polymorphisms with statistically significant differences (P9 and P10) in p300 in the interaction analysis with covariate "sex". This implied differences in haplotype distribution according to sex, and thus, the haplotype 2 (T-A) (**Table 8**) only showed significant differences in the population assigned as females at birth. The other haplotypes did not show differences in the distribution between cis and trans population, nor in males or females.

Based on experiments in rodents, it is believed that male sexual differentiation of the brain is caused by androgens, after conversion to estrogens by the aromatase. Moreover, observations in human subjects show that the direct effects of testosterone on the developing fetal brain and also during puberty, are of great importance for the development of male gender identity [43]. However, the analysis of the androgen coactivator NCOA-4 did not show any significant data.

Currently, it is still very difficult to interconnect molecular, brain, and behavioral findings [44] due to the complex interactions among behavior, genes, hormones, receptors and enzymes. But we must point out that MRI studies in people with GI, show characteristic brain profiles [5]. Both trans populations (females and males) share some common features: firstly, the involvement of the two ERs in neurobiological origin [21] and, secondly, their cortex, in some regions, is thicker than in cismen [5]. These observations support the hypothesis that transmen and transwomen undergo an atypical developmental process with respect to the sexual differentiation of their cortex [5], hypothetically, under the influence of brain estrogens, androgens, their receptors and some of their coactivators.

4.4 Consistency of the findings with the current hypothesis of a multiplicity of mechanisms involved in the complex "mosaic" model of the mammalian brain

Finally, our data are also consistent with the current hypothesis about the existence of a complex "mosaic" model of the mammalian brain [45], with a multiplicity of mechanisms involved, allowing a variable degree of masculinization/feminization within the brain. The simple model according to which testosterone masculinizes the brain of men away from a predetermined female profile, has been replaced by a complex model, according to which sexual effects on the brains of women and men are exerted by a complex combination of behavior, genetic, epigenetic and hormonal factors [45].

5. Conclusions

Based on the data presented here, we believe that it can be stated that there is a genetic basis for GI. Thus, the coactivators, NCOA-1, NCOA-2 and p300-CREBBP could be considered as candidates for increasing the list of potential "susceptibility" genes for GI. Furthermore, our data continue to support the hypothesis that GI is a multifactorial complex trait, involving intricate interactions among genes, steroids, steroids receptors and coactivators.

Acknowledgements

This work was supported by grants: ED431B 019/02 (EP), PGC2018-094919-B-C21 (AG), PGC2018-094919-B-C22 (RF, EP). We are grateful to everyone who contributed to the study, and to the trans and cis individuals who participated in particular.

Conflict of interest

The authors declare no conflict of interest.

Author details

Rosa Fernández[1*], Karla Ramírez[1,2], Enrique Delgado-Zayas[1], Esther Gómez-Gil[3], Isabel Esteva[4], Antonio Guillamon[5] and Eduardo Pásaro[1]

1 Department of Psychology, Advanced Scientific Research Center (CICA), University of A Coruña (UDC), A Coruña, Spain

2 Laboratory of Neurophysiology, Center for Biophysics and Biochemistry, Venezuelan Institute for Scientific Research (IVIC), Caracas, Bolivarian Republic of Venezuela

3 Psychiatry Service, Institute of Neurosciences, Gender Identity Unit, Hospital Clínic IDIBAPS, Barcelona, Spain

4 Endocrinology Service, Gender Identity Unit, Regional University Hospital of Málaga, Málaga, Spain

5 Department of Psychobiology, Faculty of Psychology, National University of Distance Education, Madrid, Spain

*Address all correspondence to: rosa.fernandez@udc.es

References

[1] Human Rights Campaign. Glossary of terms. http://www.hrc.org/resources/glossary-of-terms. n.d.

[2] Gómez-Gil E. Disforia de género. In: Castelo-Branco C, Molero F, editors. Manual de Sexología Clínica, Ed Médica Panamericana. 2019. p. 400–402.

[3] American Psychiatric Association. Diagnostic and Statistical Manual of Mental Disorders, 5th ed. DSM-5. Washington, DC: 2013.

[4] World Health Organization. The ICD-11. International Statistical Classification of Diseases and Related Health Problems, 11th revision (ICD-11). 2018. Available at: https://icd.who.int/browse11/l-m/en.

[5] Guillamón A, Junqué C, Gómez-Gil E. A review of the status of brain structure research in transsexualism. Arch Sex Behav. 2016;45:1615–1648. DOI: 10.1007/s10508-016-0768-5.

[6] Nguyen HB, Loughead J, Lipner E, Hantsoo L, Kornfield SL, Epperson CN. What has sex got to do with it? The role of hormones in the transgender brain. Neuropsychopharmacology. 2019;44:22–37. DOI: 10.1038/s41386-018-0140-7.

[7] Sánchez FJ and Vilain E. Genes and brain sex differences. In: Ivanka S editor. Sex Differences in the Human Brain. Their Underpinnings and Implications. Academic Press. 2010. p. 63–76. DOI: 10.1016/B978-0-444-53630-3.00005-1.

[8] Sibug R, Küppers E, Beyer C, Maxson SC, Pilgrim C, Reisert I. Genotype-dependent sex differentiation of dopaminergic neurons in primary cultures of embryonic mouse brain. Brain Res Dev Brain Res. 1996;93:136–142. DOI: 10.1016/0165-3806(96)00024-7.

[9] Lephart ED. A review of brain aromatase cytochrome P450. Brain Res Brain Res Rev. 1996;22:1–26. DOI: 10.1016/S0165-0173(96)00002-1.

[10] Kuiper GG, Carlsson B, Grandien K, Enmark E, Häggblad J, Nilsson S, et al. Comparison of the ligand binding specificity and transcript tissue distribution of estrogen receptors alpha and beta. Endocrinology. 1997;138:863–870. DOI: 10.1210/endo.138.3.4979.

[11] Henningsson S, Westberg L, Nilsson S, Lundstrom B, Ekselius L, Bodlund O, et al. Sex steroid-related genes and male-to-female transsexualism. Psychoneuroendocrinology. 2005;30:657–664. DOI: 10.1016/j.psyneuen.2005.02.006.

[12] Hare L, Bernard P, Sánchez FJJ, Baird PNN, Vilain E, Kennedy T, et al. Androgen receptor repeat length polymorphism associated with male-to-female transsexualism. Biol Psychiatry. 2009;65:93–96. DOI: 10.1016/j.biopsych.2008.08.033.

[13] Ujike H, Otani K, Nakatsuka M, Ishii K, Sasaki A, Oishi T, et al. Association study of gender identity disorder and sex hormone-related genes. Prog Neuropsychopharmacol Biol Psychiatry. 2009;33:1241–1244. DOI: 10.1016/j.pnpbp.2009.07.008.

[14] Fernández R, Esteva I, Gómez-Gil E, Rumbo T, Almaraz MC, Roda E, et al. The (CA)n polymorphism of ERβ gene is associated with FtM transsexualism. J Sex Med. 2014;11:720–728. DOI: 10.1111/jsm.12398.

[15] Foreman M, Hare L, York K, Balakrishnan K, Sánchez FJ, Harte F, et al. Genetic Link Between Gender Dysphoria and Sex Hormone Signaling. J Clin Endocrinol Metab. 2019;104:390–396. DOI: 10.1210/jc.2018-01105.

[16] Fernández R, Esteva I, Gómez-Gil E, Rumbo T, Almaraz M, Roda E, et al. Association study of ERβ, AR, and CYP19A1 genes and MtF transsexualism. J Sex Med. 2014;11: 2986–2994. DOI: 10.1111/jsm.12673.

[17] Cortés-Cortés J, R, Teijeiro N, Gómez-Gil E, Esteva I, Almaraz MC, et al. Genotypes and Haplotypes of the Estrogen Receptor α Gene (ESR1) Are Associated With Female-to-Male Gender Dysphoria. J Sex Med. 2017;14:464–472. DOI: 10.1016/j.jsxm.2016.12.234.

[18] Fernández R, Delgado-Zayas E, Ramírez K, Cortés-Cortés J, Gómez-Gil E, Esteva I, et al. Analysis of Four Polymorphisms Located at the Promoter of the Estrogen Receptor Alpha ESR1 Gene in a Population With Gender Incongruence. Sex Med. 2020;8:490–500. DOI: 10.1016/j.esxm.2020.04.002.

[19] Bentz E, Hefler L, Kaufmann U, Huber J, Kolbus A, Tempfer C. A polymorphism of the CYP17 gene related to sex steroid metabolism is associated with female-to-male but not male-to-female transsexualism. Fertil Steril. 2008;90:56–59. DOI: 10.1016/j.fertnstert.2007.05.056.

[20] Fernández R, Cortés-Cortés J, Esteva I, Gómez-Gil E, Almaraz MC, Lema E, et al. The CYP17 MspA1 Polymorphism and the Gender Dysphoria. J Sex Med. 2015;12:1329–1333. DOI: 10.1111/jsm.12895.

[21] Fernández R, Guillamon A, Cortés-Cortés J, Gómez-Gil E, Jácome A, Esteva I, et al. Molecular basis of Gender Dysphoria: androgen and estrogen receptor interaction. Psychoneuroendocrinology. 2018;98: 161–167. DOI: 10.1016/j.psyneuen.2018.07.032.

[22] Kurian JR, Olesen KM, Auger AP. Sex Differences in Epigenetic Regulation of the Estrogen Receptor-α Promoter within the Developing Preoptic Area. Endocrinology. 2010; 151:2297–2305. DOI: 10.1210/en.2009-0649.

[23] Fernández R, Ramírez K, Gómez-Gil E, Cortés-Cortés J, Mora M, Aranda G, et al. Gender-Affirming Hormone Therapy Modifies the CpG Methylation Pattern of the ESR1 Gene Promoter After Six Months of Treatment in Transmen. J Sex Med. 2020;17:1795–1806. DOI: 10.1016/j.jsxm.2020.05.027.

[24] Aranda G, Fernández-Rebollo E, Pradas-Juni M, Hanzu FA, Kalko SG, Halperin I, et al. Effects of sex steroids on the pattern of methylation and expression of the promoter region of estrogen and androgen receptors in people with gender dysphoria under cross-sex hormone treatment. J Steroid Biochem Mol Biol. 2017;172:20–28. DOI: 10.1016/j.jsbmb.2017.05.010.

[25] Métivier R, Penot G, Hübner MR, Reid G, Brand H, Kos M, et al. Estrogen receptor-alpha directs ordered, cyclical, and combinatorial recruitment of cofactors on a natural target promoter. Cell. 2003;115:751–763. DOI: 10.1016/s0092-8674(03)00934-6.

[26] Klinge CM. Estrogen receptor interaction with co-activators and co-repressors. Steroids. 2000;65:227–251. DOI: 10.1016/s0039-128x(99)00107-5.

[27] Nilsson S, Mäkelä S, Treuter E, Tujague M, Thomsen J, Andersson G, et al. Mechanisms of estrogen action. Physiol Rev. 2001;81:1535–1565. DOI: 10.1152/physrev.2001.81.4.1535.

[28] Kenna NJMC, Lanz RB, Malley BWO. Nuclear Receptor Coregulators: Cellular and Molecular Biology. Endocr Rev. 2015;20:321–344. DOI: 10.1210/edrv.20.3.0366.

[29] Cui J, Shen Y, Li R. Estrogen synthesis and signaling pathways during aging: from periphery to brain. Trends

Mol Med. 2013;19:197–209. DOI: 10.1016/j.molmed.2012.12.007.

[30] McCarthy MM. The two faces of estradiol: effects on the developing brain. Neuroscientist. 2009;15:599–610. DOI: 10.1177/1073858409340924.

[31] González M, Cabrera-Socorro A, Pérez-García CG, Fraser JD, López FJ, Alonso R, et al. Distribution patterns of estrogen receptor alpha and beta in the human cortex and hippocampus during development and adulthood. J Comp Neurol. 2007;503:790–802. DOI: 10.1002/cne.21419.

[32] Österlund MK, Gustafsson J-Å, Keller E, Hurd YL. Estrogen receptor beta (ERbeta) messenger ribonucleic acid (mRNA) expression within the human forebrain: distinct distribution pattern to ERalpha mRNA. J Clin Endocrinol Metab. 2000;85:3840–3846. DOI: 10.1210/jcem.85.10.6913.

[33] Kraus WLEE, Manning ET, Kadonaga JT. Biochemical Analysis of Distinct Activation Functions in p300 That Enhance Transcription Initiation with Chromatin Templates. Mol Cell Biol. 1999;19:8123–8135. DOI: 10.1128/mcb.19.12.8123.

[34] Wåhlin-Jacobsen S, Flanagan JN, Pedersen AT, Kristensen E, Arver S, Giraldi A. Androgen Receptor Polymorphism and Female Sexual Function and Desire. J Sex Med. 2018;15:1537–1546. DOI: 10.1016/j.jsxm.2018.09.013.

[35] Yi P, Wang Z, Chiu W, Malley BWO, Yi P, Wang Z, et al. Structure of a Biologically Active Estrogen Receptor- Coactivator Complex on DNA. Mol Cell. 2015;57:1047–1058. DOI: 10.1016/j.molcel.2015.01.025.

[36] Moore CL, Dou H, Juraska JM. Maternal stimulation affects the number of motor neurons in a sexually dimorphic nucleus of the lumbar spinal cord. Brain Res. 1992;572:52–56. DOI: 10.1016/0006-8993(92)90449-j.

[37] Eyster KM. The Estrogen Receptors : An Overview from Different Perspectives. Methods Mol Biol. 2016; 1366:1–10. DOI: 10.1007/978-1-4939-3127-9.

[38] Yore MA, Im D, Webb LK, Zhao Y, Chadwick JG, Haidacher SJ, et al. Steroid Receptor Coactivator-2 Expression In Brain And Physical Associations With Steroid Receptors. Neuroscience. 2010;169:1017–1028. DOI: 10.1016/j.neuroscience.2010.05.053.

[39] Molenda-Figueira HA, Murphy SD, Shea KL, Siegal NK, Zhao Y, Chadwick JGJ, et al. Steroid receptor coactivator-1 from brain physically interacts differentially with steroid receptor subtypes. Endocrinology. 2008;149:5272–5279. DOI: 10.1210/en.2008-0048.

[40] Auger AP, Tetel MJ, McCarthy MM. Steroid receptor coactivator-1 (SRC-1) mediates the development of sex-specific brain morphology and behavior. Proc Natl Acad Sci. 2002;97:7551–7555. DOI: 10.1073/pnas.97.13.7551.

[41] Yang XJ, Ogryzko V V, Nishikawa J, Howard BH, Nakatani Y. A p300/CBP-associated factor that competes with the adenoviral oncoprotein E1A. Nature. 1996;382:319–324. DOI: 10.1038/382319a0.

[42] Kraus WL, Kadonaga JT. p300 and estrogen receptor cooperatively activate transcription via differential enhancement of initiation and reinitiation. Genes Dev. 1998;12:331–342. DOI: 10.1101/gad.12.3.331.

[43] Swaab DF. Sexual differentiation of the human brain: relevance for gender identity, transsexualism and sexual orientation. Gynecol Endocrinol 2004;

19:301–12.DOI: 10.1080/09513590400018231.

[44] Swift-Gallant A, Monks DA. Androgenic mechanisms of sexual differentiation of the nervous system and behavior. Front Neuroendocrinol. 2017;46:32–45. DOI: 10.1016/j.yfrne.2017.04.003.

[45] Joel D, Garcia-Falgueras A, Swaab D. The Complex Relationships between Sex and the Brain. Neurosci a Rev J Bringing Neurobiol Neurol Psychiatry. 2020;26:156–169. DOI: 10.1177/1073858419867298.

Chapter 8

Consequences of Chronic Stress on the PINE Network

Verena Nold and Kelly Allers

Abstract

Stress is a risk factor for the development and progression of a variety of disorders. At the same time stress is essential to initiate adaptation to the current situation and to promote survival of the fittest. Thus, responses to stress evolved to be fast and efficient. This is implemented by a tight networking of the psycho-immune-neuro-energy (PINE) system. Within the PINE network, glucocorticoids are the universal messengers that regulate overall physiology jointly with cytokines, neurotransmitters and energy status. While the secretion of glucocorticoids in response to stress is itself a rather unspecific reaction to any kind of stressor, complexity of the outcome is encoded by lifetime, recent and present events. Together, these individual experiences modulate the diurnal and ultradian rhythmicity of glucocorticoid levels. Given the time- and dose-dependency of glucocorticoid signaling, this rhythmicity allows for flexibility in the coping with stress. In a chronic stress setting, the interaction of PINE network components is altered. While stress-resilient individuals retain adaptive capacity, vulnerable individuals lose flexibility in their responsiveness. Gene × environment interactions could explain individual differences. To better elucidate the molecular underpinnings of risk and resiliency, models that allow studying the consequences of chronic stress on the PINE network are required.

Keywords: plasticity, bioenergetics, inflammation, kynurenine pathway, glucocorticoid rhythmicity, animal model, stress, Fkbp5

1. Introduction

In the past years, the incidence of psychiatric disorders increased. Meanwhile, the majority of absence from work due to illness is attributable to psychiatric disorders. This not only impairs the affected individual but also puts a strong financial pressure on health systems [1]. Commonly, psychiatric disorders are described, classified and treated based on phenotypic symptoms. However, the success of this approach is limited since our understanding of the mechanisms leading to psychiatric pathology is far from complete and explanations to all facets of the disease remain to be discovered [2]. A first starting point to better elucidate the etiology of psychiatric disorders and to offer new treatment options is to better understand the impact of life events on physiology. These environmental influences are known to proceed onset of pathology, and together with some level of genetic susceptibility can alter brain function and overall physiology. Chronic stress is one such environmental factor and is considered a common trigger of psychiatric disorders [3]. Thus, an improved understanding of the phenomenon of stress and its consequences on physiology will support the discovery of novel treatment options or even preventive strategies. At its core, the chronic or acute inability of an individual to cope with any demand produces stress. This generic definition of stress as a response to unmet requirements proposed by Hans Selye introduces the need of responding to an adverse situation to resolve the stress exerted on the affected individual. The triggers of stress can be internal or external in nature. All non-specific reactions of the body to allow coping with challenges can be summarized under the umbrella term 'stress response'. First, an instantaneous 'fight or flight' reaction mediated by beta-adrenergic signaling introduces a shift from anabolic and restorative processes towards catabolic and energy consuming processes. Secondly, effects of hypothalamic–pituitary–adrenal axis (HPA-axis, used abbreviations are listed in 8) activation come into play to support this potential increase in energy expenditure and coordinate longer-termed stress responses. Glucocorticoids (GCs) are the messengers of this phase of stress response. They are secreted from the adrenal glands to fulfill their eponymous actions on blood glucose levels. In addition, glucocorticoid effects involve the mobilization of fatty acids and amino acids, maintenance of a sufficient blood flow to distribute nutrients and oxygen, the induction of functional changes in mitochondrial dynamics, alertness of the immune system and processing of cues in the central nervous system (CNS). In sum, these actions guarantee the necessary supply of vital tissues with adenosine-tri-phosphate (ATP) to fuel the stress response and to ultimately promote survival. After resolving the stressful situation, the HPA-axis is turned down via a negative feedback loop. Furthermore, alterations in metabolism are reverted and restoration of the emptied energy depots, healing of wounds, and mental processing of the experienced situation takes place. The body returns back to homeostasis, a term coined by Walter Bradford Cannon that translates to 'stability through constancy'. However, if certain stressors occur repeatedly, a change to these default settings might be more cost-efficient. Such a training effect can result in permanent adaptation. This process is termed allostasis, from the greek 'stability through change'. Both, the high flexibility to cope with several stressors and the ability to adapt to them were of evolutionary advantage, since less fit individuals were eliminated. Thus, an efficient and tight networking of systems required for homostasis and allostasis evolved, of which the psycho-immune-neuro-energy (PINE) network is part of.

2. Glucocorticoids are universal messengers in the PINE network

2.1 Glucocorticoids have multiple modes of action

Signaling of the HPA-axis mutually effects the metabolism, CNS, autonomous nervous system and the immune system. This is implemented by pleiotropic actions of glucocorticoids via multiple modes of actions, including non-genomic and genomic components allowing them to exert power on manifold processes. As an example for non-genomic mode of action, intercalation of GCs with plasma and mitochondrial membranes and interaction with membrane-associated receptors has been described, which enables fast-forward reactions [4]. Furthermore, GCs can trigger other non-genomic effects via their target receptors, the mineralocorticoid receptor (MR) and glucocorticoid receptor (GR) since these can interfere with cytoplasmic signaling complexes. In the medium-term, the genomic effects of glucocorticoids come into play, which are mediated by both nuclear receptors. Upon ligand binding, they translocate into the nucleus to interact with other transcription factors for example at glucocorticoid response elements (GRE) in the DNA to transactivate or transrepress a multitude of targets (reviewed in [5]. While GR and MR are ubiquitously expressed, the actual response to GCs varies widely [6].

In light of the high number of genes that is directly or indirectly affected by GR-mediated signaling, this illustrates that a tight regulation of GC signaling is present. At cellular level, this regulation is partly implemented via receptor maturation and

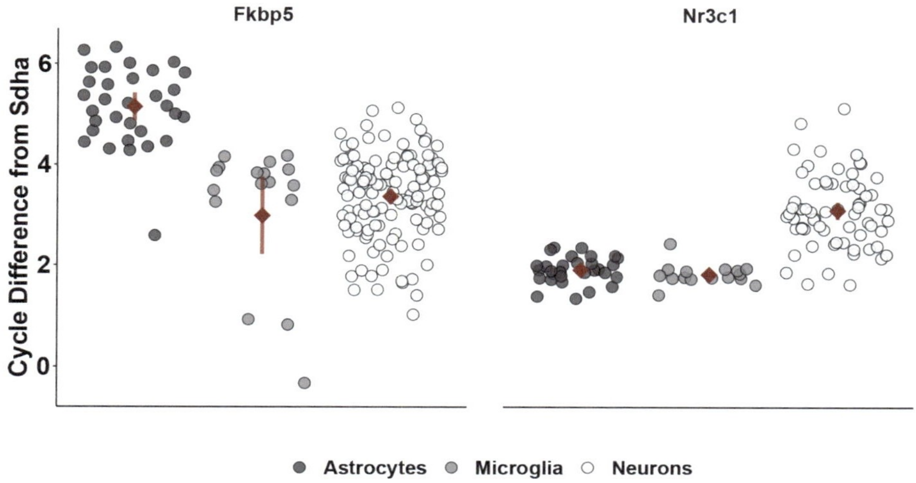

Figure 1.
Experimental details – Primary Cell Culture: *Neuronal cultures were obtained from single cell suspensions of cortex and hippocampus of embryos at E16.5. Cells were seeded in a density of 100,000 cells per 24-well and cultured at 37°C and 5% CO_2 using serum-free neurobasal medium (Invitrogen #12348017) supplemented with Glutamate, SM1 (Stemcell Technologies, Köln, Germany, #05711) and HEPES (Sigma Aldrich, Taufkirchen, Germany, #83264-100ML-F). Conditioned medium exchanges were performed every 3–4 days. On in vitro day 12 neurons were subjected to analyses. Adherent glial flask cultures were derived from enzymatically and mechanically homogenated cortices of neonates. In the culture flasks (75cm² flasks coated with Poly-L-Ornithin Hydrobromid (MW: ≤ 30,000–70,000 Dalton, Sigma #P3655)) the advanced DMEM (Invitrogen #12491015) was supplemented with HEPES, antibiotics and 10% fetal calf serum. Every 3–4 days after 1 week of flask culture, microglia were shaken off and plated at a density of 150,000 cells per 24-well of uncoated PRIMARIA plates (Corning, Germany, #353847) and analyzed in experiments the following day. For plating of astrocytes, flasks after microglia harvest were washed and the astrocyte layer was detached using 0.05% trypsin–EDTA solution (Invitrogen #25300054). Astrocytes were suspended in 50 ml advanced DMEM containing 10% FCS to stop trypsination. This suspension was used to seed the astrocytes into 24-well PRIMARIA plates (1 ml per well). On the next day, a full medium exchange was performed. On post plating day (PPD) 8 the confluent astrocyte layer was treated with AraC-medium (Cytosine Arabinoside, Sigma, #251010, 8μM) for 4 days. On PPD11, the medium was exchanged to LME-medium (L-leucine methyl esters, Sigma, #L1002, 50 mM) for 1 hour and astrocytes were subsequently washed three times with medium. On PPD14, the medium was exchanged to serum-free medium and the assay was performed the next day.* ***Experimental details – qPCR:*** *Native or stimulated cells were lysed in 250μl RLT buffer (Qiagen, Hilden, Germany, #79216) containing 1% beta-mercapto-ethanol (Sigma #M3148-100ML) and frozen at −80°C prior to RNA isolation. RNA was isolated using RNeasy Plus kit (Qiagen #74192) following the manufacturer's recommendations. Integrity was confirmed to be RIN > 8 (Fragmentanalyser, Thermo Fisher Scientific, Langenselbold, Germany). For normalization, 500 ng of total mRNA were used during reverse transcription (high capacity cDNA kit, Qiagen #4368813). All TaqMan gene expression assays were labeled with FAM (Thermo Fisher #4352042; succinate dehydrogenase complex subunit A (Sdha, Mm01352366_m1), murine Fkbp5 (Mm00487403_m1), glucocorticoid receptor (Nr3c1, Mm00433832_m1)) and used in conjunction with the fast universal PCR Master Mix (Thermo Fisher #4351368). Samples were analyzed in technical triplicates on a QuantStudio 6 (Thermo Fisher). All gene expression levels were normalized within the same cell type relative to the cycle thresholds measured for Sdha and for stimulation experiments relative to DMSO-treated cells.* ***Results:*** *Primary murine astrocytes, microglia and neurons differ in their basal mRNA expression of the glucocorticoid receptor (Nr3c1) and its functional inhibitor FK506 binding protein 51 (Fkbp5). Analysis of qPCR cycle number difference from housekeeper (Sdha) revealed that cell types differed in the expression of Fkbp5 ($F(3, 168) = 33.5; p < .0001$) which post hoc was attributable to astrocytes displaying the lowest expression of Fkbp5 compared to microglia and neurons. Nr3c1 was higher expressed in both glial cell types compared to neurons (Kruskal-Wallis rank sum test $\chi^2(3) = 64.1, p < .0001$). Individual data points are shown alongside with their mean ± 95% confidence interval (red). Shades of gray indicate the cell type: astrocytes (dark gray, left), microglia (gray, middle) and neurons (ecru, right). High values in the PCR cycles needed to reach the set threshold represent low amounts of the targeted mRNA and hence a low expression of the gene while low cycle numbers indicate higher expression.*

turn over. In the cytoplasm, the functioning of the GR is modulated by a molecular hetero-complex that comprises heat shock proteins (HSP), protein phosphatases and a number of co-chaperones. The immunophilin FK506-binding protein 51 FKBP51, encoded by the FKBP5 gene, is one of them. This co-chaperone functionally inhibits glucocorticoid signaling by interfering with the maturation of the glucocorticoid receptor complex. If the GR-HSP90 complex is bound to FKBP51, the

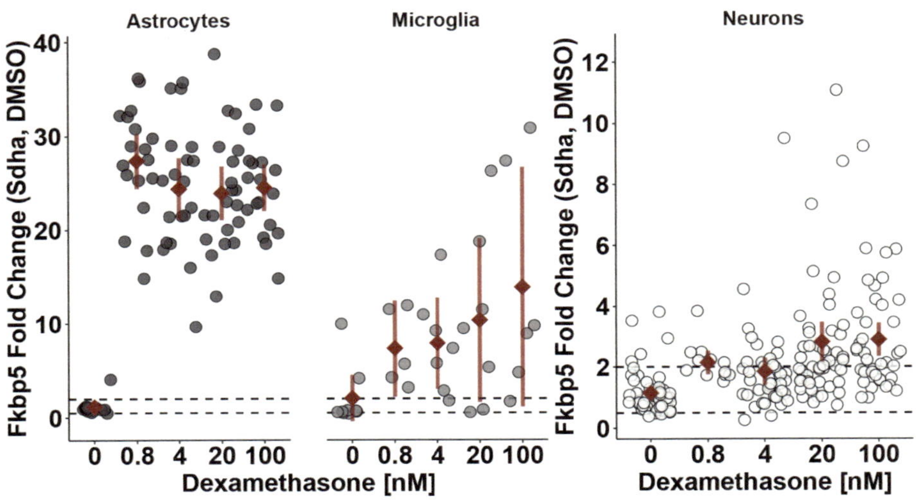

Figure 2.
*Cells were cultured and RNA analyses were performed as described in **Figure 1. Experimental details – Glucocorticoid Stimulation:** Stocks of dexamethasone solved in dimethyl sulfoxide (DMSO) were freshly diluted 1:200 in warmed culture medium. Cells were stimulated by replacing 0.5 ml of the medium with the obtained dexamethasone dilutions so that final concentrations of 0.8, 4, 20 or 100 nM were applied. Stimulation was performed between 08:00 a.m. to 10:00 a.m. for 4 hours. To control for manipulation or vehicle effects, a half medium exchange was performed or cells were treated with medium containing 0.005% DMSO, respectively. **Results:** Stimulation with increasing doses of the synthetic glucocorticoid dexamethasone elicited different induction of the glucocorticoid response element harboring Fkbp5 gene, dependent of cell type and dose ($F(8, 309) = 95.9$, $p < .0001$). Astrocytes (dark gray) showed a stronger induction than microglia (gray), while neurons (ecru) were not responsive. Individual data points are shown alongside with their mean ± 95% confidence interval (red).*

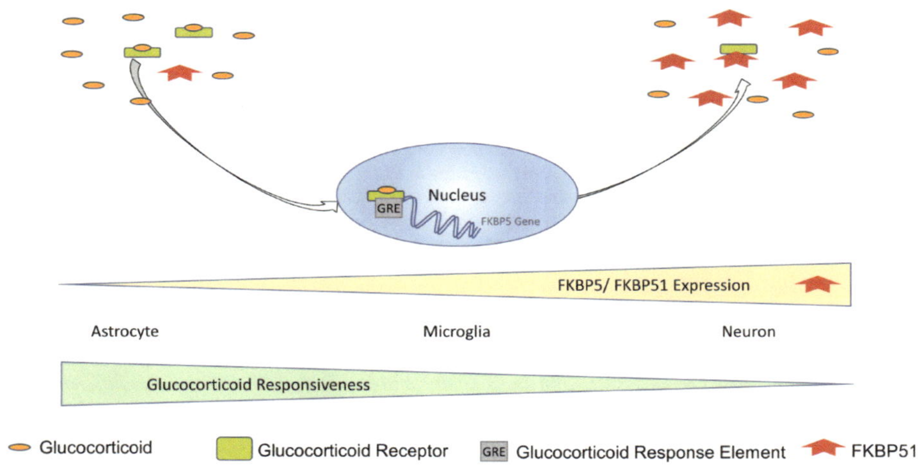

Figure 3.
Mechanistic overview of the interaction between Fkbp5 expression and GC abundancy on GC-induced gene transcription.

GR is in a low affinity state [7]. With these altered dissociation kinetics, more ligand, more GRs or a longer time is needed in order to elicit the same amount of nuclear translocations of the GR as in the presence of fewer FKBP51 molecules. Thus, the abundance of GR and FKBP51 influences the cellular responsivity to GCs and is part of the cellular identity [8]. In the CNS, astrocytes and microglia express the GR at comparable levels, but more than neurons. Astrocytes were found to

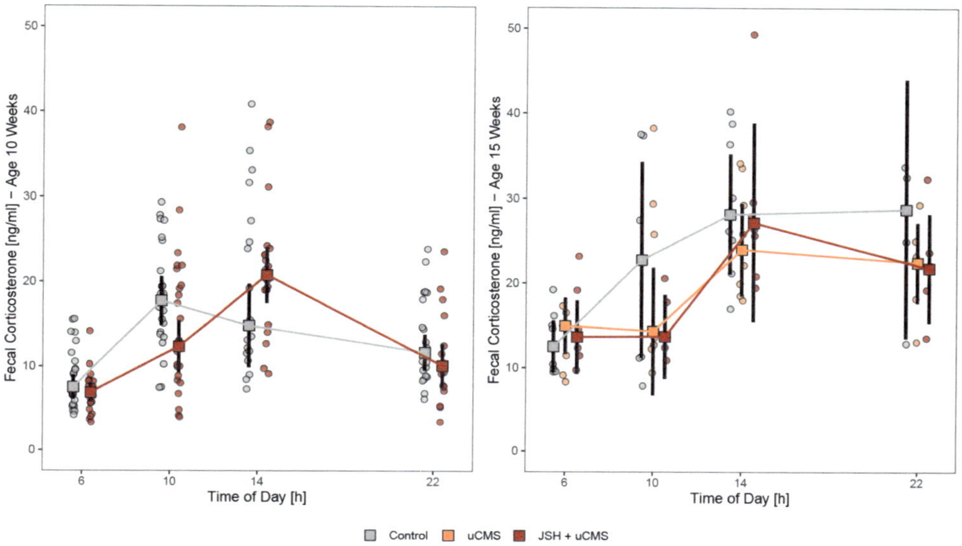

Figure 4.
Experimental details - uCMS: *Test-naïve male Wistar Kyoto rats were obtained from Charles River at an age of 5 weeks and randomly assigned into the experimental groups. All experiments were performed under an inverse 12 hour light cycle (sunrise 18:00, sunset 6:00 with a ramp of 30 minutes). Controls were housed in groups of three throughout the experiment and were sheltered from olfactory, visual or acoustic cues of the stress rats by a Scantainer (Scanbur, Denmark). Rats assigned to the uCMS group were housed in groups of 3 until an age of 10 weeks while uCMS + JSH animals were single housed upon the day of arrival. From an age of 10 weeks onwards, the uCMS protocol started. Only mild stressors such as wet bedding, frequent changes of the bedding, timely limited food and water restriction, intruder confinements, reduction of provided space and flashing lights were applied. Experiments were carried out in male Wistar Kyoto rats under allowance of the regional council for animal welfare (Regierungspräsidium Tübingen, Baden-Württemberg, Germany) and in compliance with directive 2020/63/EU.* ***Experimental details – Corticosterone:*** *Feces samples were collected directly from the animals at 6 a.m., 10 a.m., 2 p.m. and 10 p.m. on the same day and lyophilized. From 50 mg powder of each sample ethanolic extracts were obtained. After evaporation of the ethanol, samples were resuspended in assay buffer and a competitive enzyme-linked immune assay (Cayman Chemicals, Ann Arbor, Michigan, USA) was performed following the manufacturer's instructions. Individual data points are visualized alongside the mean ± the 95% confidence interval.* ***Results:*** *Diurnal Rhythm of Corticosterone Measured in Feces of Rats exposed to Unpredictable Chronic Mild Stress (uCMS) in Young Adulthood with or without Prior Juvenile Single Housing (JSH) in Comparison to Controls.* ***Left:*** *After 5 weeks of JSH the diurnal rhythm of corticosterone was traced in feces of control (gray) and single housed rats (red). Type III sum of square ANOVA of the linear mixed effect model of group-by-time effect corrected for the random effect of each individual animal indicated a significant effect of time ($\chi^2(3) = 92, p < .00001$) and group ($\chi^2(1) = 3.9, p = .048$). Post hoc tests revealed differences between controls and JSH at 10:00 ($t(169) = 1.97, p = .05$). Moreover, in JSH rats a clear peak in corticosterone was observed at 2 p.m. when levels were significantly different from 6 a.m. ($t(135) = 7.3, p < .0001$), 10 a.m. ($t(127) = 3.6, p < .003$) and 10 p.m. ($t(134) = 5, p < .0001$), while between 6 a.m. and 10 a.m. the levels already increased significantly ($t(129) = 4.1, p = .0004$). However in controls, the peak was observed earlier at 10 a.m. and levels slowly decreased over noon. This was reflected by significant differences between 6 a.m. and 10 a.m. ($t(130) = 5.1, p <.0001$), 2 p.m. ($t(133) = 5.3, p < .0001$) as well as 11 p.m. and the 10 a.m. ($t(128) = 2.8, p = .03$) and 2 p.m. ($t(137) = 3.1, p = .01$).* ***Right:*** *After 5 weeks of uCMS alone (peach) or in addition to JSH (red), the diurnal corticosterone rhythm was traced in feces and revealed a similar pattern for both stress groups that differed from the pattern in controls (gray). While in controls the levels increased over the morning and noon leading to a peak in the afternoon (6 a.m. vs. 2 p.m. $t(53) = 4$, $p = .001$; 10 p.m. vs. 6 a.m. $t(59) = 2.6, p = .056$), in the stress groups the levels between 6 a.m. and 10 a.m. remained the same, peaked in the afternoon (uCMS: $t(55) = 2.8, p = .03$; uCMS + JSH: $t(55) = 4.1$, $p = .0007$) and began to decrease again towards the night.*

express lower levels of FKBP5 than microglia and neurons, which upon GC-stimulation resulted in a stronger responsiveness of astrocytes, followed by microglia and neurons (**Figures 1–3** modified from [8]). This indicates that abundance of GR relative to FKBP51 imparts a cell-type specific fine tuning of the GC response magnitude at a given time. In addition, this ratio is modulated by recent fluctuations in GC exposure. These modulations are essential for proper functioning [9, 10].

2.2 Origins of dynamic glucocorticoid flows

The exposure of cells to GCs relies on the activity of the HPA-axis. Once triggered, neurosecretory nerve terminals within the hypothalamic paraventricular nucleus are activated to release corticotropin-releasing hormone (CRH) into the portal system of the anterior pituitary, where in response, adreno-cortico-tropic hormone (ACTH) is secreted, transported across the blood–brain-barrier into the peripheral circulation and in the adrenal glands to stimulate the secretion of glucocorticoids into the blood. Over the course of the day, the levels of glucocorticoids undergo substantial fluctuations. While in man cortisol levels peak in the morning, in nocturnal animals like laboratory rodents nadir levels are observed in the morning. Chronic exposure to stress triggers changes in the pattern of this diurnal rhythmicity i.e. shifts in the timing of the peak (**Figure 4** modified from [11]). Besides the diurnal pattern, ultradian rhythms influence the actual plasma levels [12].

These oscillations are enabled via feedback loops between components of the HPA-axis and inside each cell. The feedback occurs at different kinetics and thus introduces phase shifts. Such delays are based on differential glucocorticoid affinity and expression of MR compared to GR, episodic transcription of the rate-limiting enzymes necessary for steroidogenesis, as well as offsets between secretion and distribution of glucocorticoids. In addition, an ultra-short negative feedback loop within each cell is present, since GCs induce the transcription of their functional inhibitor FKBP5 and have the potential to shut down their own signaling [13]. Thus, FKBP5 levels can regulate cellular GC-responsiveness temporally dependent on previous fluctuations in glucocorticoid levels. This generates an additional degree of freedom and flexibility in the stress response system. Interestingly, dynamic changes of GCs are known to be required for normal emotional and cognitive reactions [10, 14]. In humans, several single-nucleotide polymorphisms (SNPs) have been described, which are associated with differential induction of FKBP5 upon glucocorticoid stimulation and thus contribute to the variability of stress perception and coping in the population [15].This illustrates that appropriate negative feedback is required to allow for diurnal and ultradian oscillations of GCs, and that attenuation of the latter goes hand in hand with altered HPA-axis responsiveness and stress coping, which ultimately can impact health. Together, the 24 hours cycle and the ultradian oscillations of GC levels are known to have strong influence on functioning of the body. For reference, the interplay of dynamic GC levels with the PINE network is described in the following sections.

2.3 Biphasic effects of glucocorticoids on the immune system

After their release from the adrenal glands, glucocorticoids are distributed throughout the body via the blood, which is not only the medium for information transportation, but also a home base of the immune system. The reactions of the immune system to glucocorticoids are known to be time-, condition- and dose-dependent. This results in several phases. As part of the fight or flight response, catecholamines are immediately released via the sympathetic-adrenal-medullary system and trigger the mobilization of monocytes from the bone marrow as a consequence of stress [16]. Glucocorticoids and catecholamines then act together in this preparatory phase with an increased perfusion of peripheral tissues ensuring the energy supply of peripheral tissues for the fight or flight response but also the distribution of the mobilized monocytes. In the event of wounding, blood can flush out pathogens and contribute to an initial sealing of the wound. During the acute phase of stress and high glucocorticoid exposure, the immune system itself is suppressed to reduce inflammation-associated swelling of tissue. Furthermore the liberated energy can be allocated for fighting the current situation rather than pathogens. In the clinic, these immunosuppressive effects of GC are widely exploited in the treatment of inflammatory diseases and autoimmune disorders. On a molecular level, this can be explained by the GC-mediated inhibition of nuclear factor kappa-light-chain-enhancer of activated B cells (NFκB) and glucocorticoid receptor signaling which is followed by a downregulation of pro-inflammatory cytokines and modulation of T-cell activity [5]. In contrast to the inhibitory effects of acute, high doses of GCs, in vitro studies suggest that low doses of GCs, which rather elicit mineralocorticoid receptor signal transduction, trigger pro-inflammatory responses in stimulated macrophages [7]. Since exposure to a stressor is potentially linked to subsequent tissue damage and contagion with bacteria or viruses, this mechanism may be implemented to gear up the immune system in preparation for the fighting of potential infections in the aftermath of stress. In addition, glucocorticoids change the expression of cell adhesion molecules on endothelial cells and immune cells. While glucocorticoid receptor signaling in response to high doses of glucocorticoids is associated with decreased expression of adhesion molecules and less extravasation of immune cells [17], mineralocorticoid receptor mediated signaling in response to decreasing GC levels is associated with higher expression of adhesion molecules that facilitates crossing of the vascular wall for immune cells [18]. Outside of the blood vessels, the formerly mobilized monocytes differentiate into tissue macrophages to clear received wounds from pathogens or destroyed cells [19] Taken together, these findings point towards a biphasic mode of action of the GC in the context of immune responses, with the exchange from acute immune suppressive effects of high dose GCs to pro-inflammatory effects as the levels of GCs decrease. Such dynamic responses to stress and glucocorticoids are also observed in other components of the PINE network.

2.4 Wiring of neural stress circuits is shaped by glucocorticoids

The brain is a highly adaptive organ and retains the ability to change throughout life via a process termed (neuro-)plasticity. In response to experiences and learning, plasticity involves the weakening or strengthening of synapses on a cellular level and circuits between brain areas on an anatomical level. Given the individuality of experiences, this results in unique wiring of the brain and could explain why stress has a different meaning for different people under different conditions. During childhood and adolescence the brain is still maturing and undergoes changes that require even more plasticity. During these developmental phases, the processing of inputs is less deterministic than in adults, which on one side enables flexible learning but on the other side puts young individuals at risk to adopt adverse stress coping and emotional processing approaches that ultimately render them more vulnerable to develop psychiatric symptoms [20]. Indeed, stress and trauma have been reported to severely damage the developing brain [21]. Comparisons of normally developed brain functionality, brains from individuals that suffered from early life adversity such as abuse or neglect, or brains of psychiatric patients revealed that a defined set of brain areas is most commonly affected by stress, namely the hippocampus, amygdala, and prefrontal cortex (PFC). These brain regions are strongly connected and their networking determines what is perceived as threat and how individuals cope with stress and adversity. Protective factors associated with adequate coping include the ability to stay optimistic, a controlled regulation of emotions, high levels of attention set shifting to focus on different aspects of the current situation, the capacity to reflect on experiences and own reactions and higher cognitive abilities required for executive functions. All of these functions are biologically linked within the network comprising the hippocampus, amygdala, and PFC. Upon perception, the medial PFC filters and processes sensory inputs to initiate thoughts and actions in accordance with internal goals, based on previously learned behaviors retrieved from the hippocampus. To orchestrate defensive physiological and behavioral responses, the PFC is connected to the amygdala, the emotion regulation area of the brain, which in turn contributes to sympathetic and HPA-axis activation and intensifies long-term memory consolidation of adverse emotional events in the hippocampus. By dampening emotions produced in the amygdala, the PFC supports maintenance of cognitive flexibility in challenging situations. This indirectly influences learning processes in the hippocampus, but the PFC can also directly dampen hippocampal signaling and thus modulate memory formation. In the context of memory formation, an inverted U-shaped association of glucocorticoid levels and plasticity has been observed. Since the modulation of cellular activity via glucocorticoids was reported to be brain region-dependent, this could indicate that differential expression of GC-responsive receptors play a role in this biphasic pattern [9]. Indeed, activation of GRs in the presence of high glucocorticoid concentrations were reported to impair long-term potentiation (LTP) by high-frequency stimulation and enhanced long-term depression. While low levels of GCs selectively activate MR signaling, which increases LTP via θ-burst stimulation and increased expression of N-methyl-d-aspartate (NMDA) receptors and thus glutamatergic, excitatory signaling. Whether potentially newly formed synapses persist to change memory and ultimately the way how future stressful events are dealt with, depends on their stability. The expression of cell adhesion molecules contributes to the synaptic stability. Like in endothelial and immune cells, glucocorticoids were found to influence the expression of glycoprotein cell-adhesion molecules in [22]. Not only their presence, but fluctuations in the levels of glucocorticoids were reported to be required for plasticity [23], which could add additional explanation why stress-associated fluctuations in GC levels have a strong influence on memory formation. Summed up, the communication of a challenging situation via glucocorticoids is handled in multiple phases, which allows for additional set screws like dose, timing and previous events to fine-tune stress responses in the brain. In the long run, changes in glucocorticoid levels and differential expression of their receptors can influence emotional, executive and cognitive responses to stress by interacting with plasticity and networking of the amygdala, PFC and hippocampus. Of note, this remodeling in response to challenges allows for adaptation to the current environment but also to adequately regulate the assessment of future challenges. Thus, a high level of plasticity is beneficial to continuously update the connectivity of these sensory-defense circuits. Dependent on individual resiliency factors and in particular contexts, stress challenges may result in personal growth regarding the balancing of anxiety, mood control, memory, and decision making. At the same time, frequent stress challenges can strengthen certain connections within the brain. This training effect might be cost-effective in steady environments, but could be maladaptive in case of persistence and lack of reversibility due to reduced plasticity. Optimizing the choice between homeostatic and allostatic processes is a complex task of the PINE network that involves consideration of associated energetic costs.

2.5 Glucocorticoids interact with mitochondria to regulate energy

Mitochondria are the main providers of energy, namely ATP. Besides glycolysis and fatty acid oxidation, the majority of ATP is produced during oxidative phosphorylation. The motor for the production of ATP is an inward rectifying proton gradient across the inner mitochondrial membrane. In the process of generating this gradient, a series of redox-reactions occurs at complex I to V of the electron transport chain (ETC), which consumes oxygen and substrates generated in the tricarboxic acid cycle [24]. According to the endosymbiont theory, mitochondria are

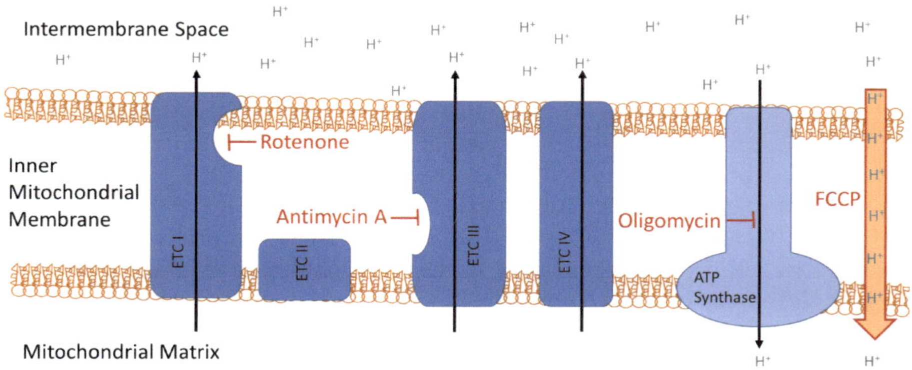

Figure 5.
Schematic of the mitochondrial electron transport chain (ETC) and the sites of action of the inhibitors and uncouplers used to study respirometric performance.

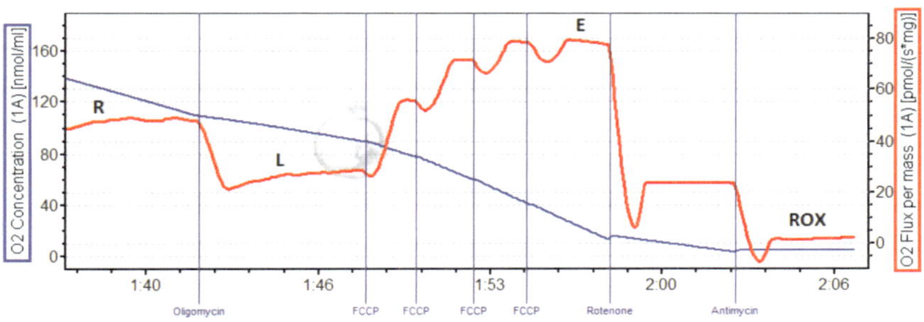

Figure 6.
Animal housing and stress protocols are described in ***Figure 4. Experimental details – High Resolution Respirometry:*** *Rats were sacrificed between 7 a.m. to 11 a.m. under deep anesthesia (intra peritoneal injection of 100 mg pentobarbital/kg body weight, Narcoren®, Boehringer Ingelheim Pharma GmbH & Co KG, Germany). The rostral halves of the right hippocampi were isolated and stored in ice-cold custodial® (DR. FRANZ KÖHLER CHEMIE GMBH, Bensheim, Germany). Immediately before respirometry, the tissue was homogenated, diluted to a concentration of 2 mg/ml with mitochondrial respiration medium MiRO5 (Oroboros Instruments, Innsbruck, Austria) and loaded into the calibrated oxygraph chambers which were pre-warmed to 37°C. Measurements were performed in duplicates. In brief, pyruvate (5 mM), glutamate (10 mM), malate (0.5 mM), cytochrome c (10 µM), ADP (5 mM) and succinate (10 mM) were added to measure routine respiration. By injecting oligomycin (2.5 µM), the ATP-sythase was inhibited and the LEAK state of respiration was induced. Next the uncoupler FCCP was titrated in steps of 0.5 µM to determine the maximal capacity of the ETC. By adding rotenone (0.5 µM), the amount of oxygen consumed independent of complex I was determined. Lastly, antimycin A (2.5 µM) as inhibitor of complex III was injected to measure the residual oxygen consumption (ROX) outside of mitochondria. All chemicals were purchased from Sigma-Aldrich (Sigma-Aldrich Company Ltd., St. Louis, Missouri, USA).* ***Results:*** *Exemplary recording of high-resolution respirometry analysis in rat hippocampal homogenate. The blue line represents the oxygen concentration measured via polarographic oxgen sensors over the course of the experiment shown in hours, while the red line indicates its first derivative, the oxygen flux. The injection of inhibitors and the titration of uncouplers of the ETC is indicated by horizontal lines and marks switches between respirometric states: R = routine, L = LEAK, E = maximal electron transfer (in the uncoupled state), ROX = residual oxygen consumption.*

remnants of bacteria which were incorporated as cell organelles into eukaryotic cells. As such, mitochondria still harbor 37 genes on their own mitochondrial DNA (mtDNA), while genes encoding other mitochondrial components were transferred to the nuclear DNA. Glucocorticoids hence can not only influence mitochondria by intercalating into their membranes or by regulating the expression of nuclear genes relevant for mitochondrial function, but also directly interfere with mtDNA in a time and dose-dependent manner [25]. These interactions guarantee a sufficient energy supply during stress. In a chronic mild stress study carried out in Wistar Kyoto rats, an adaptive activation of the ETC and higher respirometric performance was observed (**Figures 5–7**, modified from [11]). However, increased activity of the ETC leads to the production of reactive oxygen species (ROS). Complex I activity is associated with more production of ROS than complex II [26]. In a defined manner, ROS serve as important signaling molecules [27] and are essential for the oxidative burst observed in granulocytes to fight microbial infections. In higher doses, ROS can outbalance anti-oxidative defense system which results in oxidative stress [28]. In that event, proteins, lipids and DNA becomes damaged and lose functionality. Based on their microscopic structure and cellular location, mitochondria are especially vulnerable to oxidative stress [29]. In the long run, chronically elevated mitochondrial activity can thus result in a decompensation of the energy providing system. A shift away from ETC complex I towards complex II, as seen in the above cited chronic mild stress study, might be a possibility to reduce ROS overload and to evade the risk of oxidative stress. In addition to their bioenergetic role,

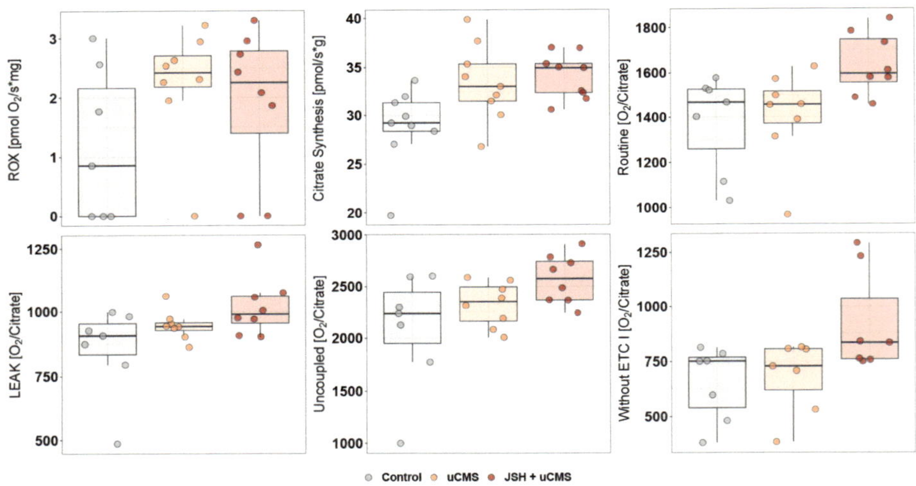

Figure 7.
Animal housing and stress protocols are described in ***Figure 4*** *while the respirometry protocol is illustrated in* ***Figure 5. Experimental details – Citrate Synthase Activity:*** *By coupling the synthesis of citrate and CoA-SH from oxalacetate and acetyl-CoA with the formation of TNB out of DTNB and CoA-SH, the activity of the citrate synthase in frozen homogenates of hippocampus samples was measured spectro-photometrically as the rate of increase in absorbance. In brief, 0.1 M triethanolamine HCl buffer, oxalacetate (10 mM), DTNB (1.01 mM) and the citrate synthase standard were freshly prepared on every experimental day. Distilled water was loaded into 1 ml glass cuvettes together with 100 µl of DTNB, 50 µl oxalacetate, 25 µl acetyl CoA and 25 µl Triton and sample or standard. The absorbance was measured at 32°C.* ***Results:*** *Comparison of the respirometric performance of permeabilized hippocampal homogenate derived from 16 weeks old controls (gray), rats that underwent 5 weeks of uCMS during young adulthood (peach) and rats that were subjected to 5 weeks of JSH prior to uCMS (red). In both stress groups, an increase in mitochondrial mass, measured via citrate synthase activity, was detected ($F(2,24) = 5.7$, $p = .009$; uCMS: $t = 2.7$, $p = .03$; JSH + uCMS: $t = 3.1$, $p = .01$). After normalization to this enzyme activity, statistically significant effects of stress on routine ($F(2,20) = 5.39$, $p = .03$) and respiration without ETC complex I ($F(2,18) = 3.7$, $p = .03$) was suggestive. Tukey's honest significant difference post-hoc testing confirmed that in the double-stress group (JSH + uCMS) compared to controls the routine respiration ($t = 2.6$, $p = .04$) and respiration without ETC complex I ($t = 2.7$, $p = .04$) was increased.*

mitochondria are involved in regulation of apoptosis and calcium homeostasis which were shown to be modulated by GC signaling [30, 31]. This contributes to their key role in regulating synaptic transmission, brain function, and cognition [32]. Taken together, mitochondria are an interesting platform for further communication of GC signaling [33]. Notably, the communication from the HPA-axis to mitochondria is not unilateral, because mitochondria are the site of glucocorticoid production. As such, they express stress-inducible translocator proteins (TSPOs) that modulate oxidative stress and transport cholesterol from the outer to the inner mitochondrial membrane [34]. In addition, mitochondria harbor enzymes required for the cleavage of nutrition-derived cholesterol into precursors of GCs as well as enzymes involved in the conversion of the inactive 11-deoxycortisol or deoxicorticosterone to the bio active cortisol and corticosterone. Thus, mitochondria regulate GC availability and are an additional set screw in the complex feedback structure of GC signaling and the stress response system.

3. The brain recaptures networking of PINE components

Given the importance of the PINE network for stress responses and health, additional ways of communication between its components in addition to GC signaling evolved. The brain is a central hub for the orchestration of stress responses. At the same time it is anatomically rather isolated from the rest of the body and thus contains highly specialized cells that generate functional output and cells that support, shape and surveil the activity in that micro model of the body. The following sections issue in more detail how these tasks are shared in the central nervous system and how chronic stress modulates this.

3.1 Microglia govern the immunity of the brain

In the brain, full blown immune reactions including sudden tissue loss would be deleterious for the fine-tuned neuronal circuits and networks. Therefore, the brain is especially protected from wounding via the skull and a tight interface of astrocytes, pericytes and endothelial cells, termed blood brain barrier, limits the access of blood-born immune responses to the brain. As replacement for the peripheral immune cells, the brain harbors specialized tissue-resident immune competent cells, the microglia. These belong to the monocyto-phagocyting-system like macrophages and are of mesenchymal origin. Besides their phagocytic properties to clear debris, microglia contribute to the pruning of synapses during development and learning. In addition, microglia have a ramified shape in the resting state and monitor the brain parenchyma for pathogen associated molecular patterns or danger associated molecular patterns. Upon detection of such patterns, microglia become activated and change towards a more amoeboid shape that allows for increased mobility. In parallel, different receptors like the cannabinoid receptor 2 or toll-like receptors become expressed on their surface to guide microglia via chemotactic signaling to the site where the activating signal originated from. Once activated, microglia proliferate and produce inflammatory cytokines like interleukin 1 β, interleukin 6 or tumor necrosis factor α. Analogous to inflammation in the periphery, these stimuli trigger clonal expansion and attract more immune cells. Normally, all immune cells in the brain are derived from a residual microglia pool, but in case of severe inflammation the blood–brain-barrier becomes leaky and other immune cells can enter the brain. The latter implies a certain neurotoxic effect of proinflammatory responses initiated by microglia. To prevent this take over from peripheral immune cells and the associated risk for loss of functional connectivity in the brain, the brain modifies behavior of an individual with potential dangerous infection, as measured by elevated pro-inflammatory cytokine levels, in such a way that the individual withdraws from demanding activities to allow allocation of more energy to fighting the source of infection. This phenomenon is termed 'cytokine induced sickness behavior' and besides altered neurotransmitter signaling, GCs are mediators of this switch that shall protect the brain from severe inflammation. Theoretically, it should also prevent the infected person from entering the general population and spreading the disease. After resolution of the inflammatory insult, returning to a normal state is essential for brain physiology. This involves apoptosis of invaded peripheral immune cells, a switchback to resting microglia or apoptosis of activated microglia as well as tightening of the blood brain barrier.

3.2 Astrocytes provide (metabolic) support to neurons

Astrocytes are an essential component of the blood brain barrier and thus play a crucial role in the protection of the CNS from peripheral cues. In addition, astrocytes regulate the flow of nutrients. This enables astrocytes to metabolically support neurons [35]. For example, astrocytes are involved in the glutamate-glutamine cycle and catabolize glucose via the tri-carboxic acid cycle, which generates lactate that is shuttled to neurons to allow them to directly perform oxidative phosphorylation. While glycolysis produces only 2 ATP molecules from one molecule glucose, oxidative phosphorylation is more efficient and produces between 30 and 36 ATP molecules, dependent on proton leakage across the mitochondrial membrane [36]. In the presence of GCs, this alternative energy source for neurons becomes especially relevant, since GCs reduce the cellular uptake of glucose and glutamate [37]. Enhanced clearance of the synaptic cleft from glutamate by astrocytes could therefore be another way to safe-guard neurons from short-comings in energy. Besides their supportive role in terms of metabolism, astrocytes were shown to influence information processing and cognition by integrating local sensory information and behavioral state [38, 39]. In response to glucocorticoids, astrocytes were reported to directly influence (emotional) learning by regulating neurogenesis and structurally reorganizing neuronal networks [40]. This is possibly due to their role in stabilizing synapses and their responsibility for the rapid clearance of the synaptic cleft. As an example, astrocytes express excitatory amino acid transporters (EAAT1–5) to remove glutamate from the synapse and furthermore recycle it for further use in neurons [41]. Astrocytes hence play an important role in shaping plasticity in response to emotional stress and set the stage for future stressful encounters [42]. In addition, glia cells can regulate neurotransmission by generating neuroactive substances. The kynurenine pathway is one example where balancing of astrocytes and microglia activity is required for adequate modulation of neuronal communication.

3.3 Interplay of CNS-cell types in the kynurenine pathway

The clear distribution of roles between neurons, microglia and astrocytes requires several sites of interaction in order to balance the different activities in the CNS. An example of these interaction points is the kynurenine pathway. The essential amino acid tryptophan is mainly catabolized via this pathway, while only a minor amount ($\sim$5%) is used up for the production of the neurotransmitter serotonin. As first step of the pathway, stress-induced GCs lead to an upregulation of the enzyme tryptophan-di-oxygenase (TDO), which converts tryptophan to kynurenine. This enzyme is mostly expressed in the liver [43]. In the brain, microglia can convert tryptophan to kynurenine via the indole-amine-di-oxygenase (IDO) enzyme, which is inducible by pro-inflammatory cytokines. Alternatively, astrocytes can shuttle peripheral kynurenine across the blood brain barrier into the CNS. From kynurenine, two neuroactive substances are produced, kynurenic acid and quinolinic acid. Under a pro-inflammatory state, microglia dominate kynurenine metabolism and process it via kynurenine-mono-oxygenase (KMO) to quinolinic acid, since KMO becomes highly expressed in the presence of pro-inflammatory cytokines. Quinolinic acid is an NMDA receptor agonist with pro-oxidative capacities. In an anti-inflammatory state, kynurenine may be processed by the astrocytic kynurenine-amino-transferases (KATs) to kynurenic acid. In contrast to quinolinic acid, kynurenic acid has anti-oxidant properties and is an NMDA receptor antagonist. Furthermore, kynurenic acid reduces the release of dopamine and glutamate [44, 45]. An astrocytic dominance of the kynurenine pathway and thus a shift to higher kynurenic acid relative to quinolinic acid thus is considered neuroprotective. However, reduced excitatory neurotransmission could result in reduced synaptic plasticity [46]. In a chronic mild stress study in rats, reduced expression of immediate early genes in the PFC, which suggests a decreased ability

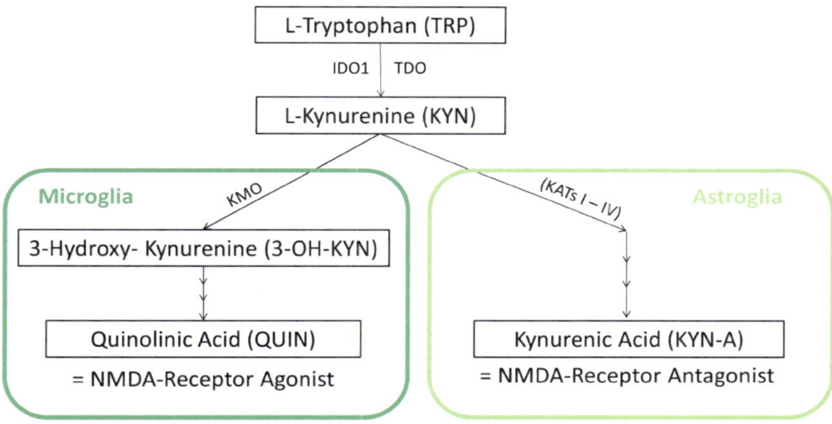

Figure 8.
Overview of trypotophan catabolism by enzymes of the kynurenine pathway in the CNS.

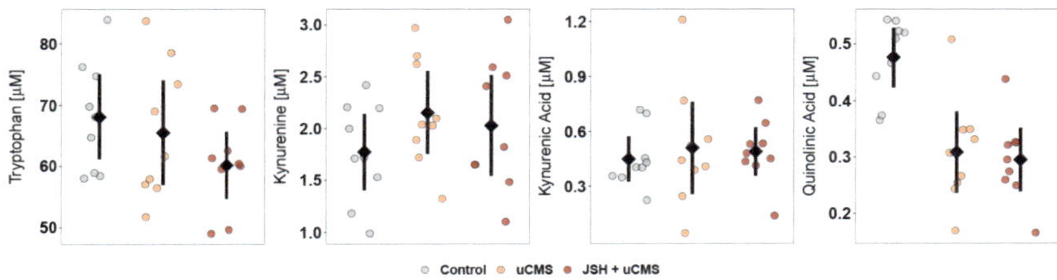

Figure 9.
Animal housing and stress protocols are described in ***Figure 4. Experimental details – HPLC-MS/MS Quantification of TRYCATs:*** *Tandem mass spectrometry (HPLC-MS/MS) was used for simultaneous quantification of tryptophan (TRP) and its catabolites kynurenic acid (KYNA), kynurenine (KYN) and quinolinic acid (QUIN) in plasma. After protein precipitation with ice-cold methanol, a reversed phase chromatography was performed followed by mass spectrometric detection in the positive ion multiple reaction monitoring mode. Deuterated analogues of the analytes, namely d5-kynurenic acid, d4-kynurenine, and d3-quinolinic acid were used as internal standards. The lower limits of quantification were 625 nM for TRP, 62.5 nM for KYN, 12.5 nM for KYNA and 25 nM for QUIN.* ***Results:*** *Activation of the kynurenine pathway in response to stress exposure. Comparison is shown between controls (gray) and rats exposed to 5 weeks of unpredictable chronic mild stress in adutlhood (peach) as well as rats subjected to 5 weeks of juvenile single housing (JSH) prior to uCMS (red). Data point represent individual animals and are shown alongside with the mean ± 95% confidence interval. In both stress groups, the levels of the NMDA receptor agonist quinolinic acid were significantly decreased compared to controls ($F(2,24) = 14.4$, $p = .0001$).*

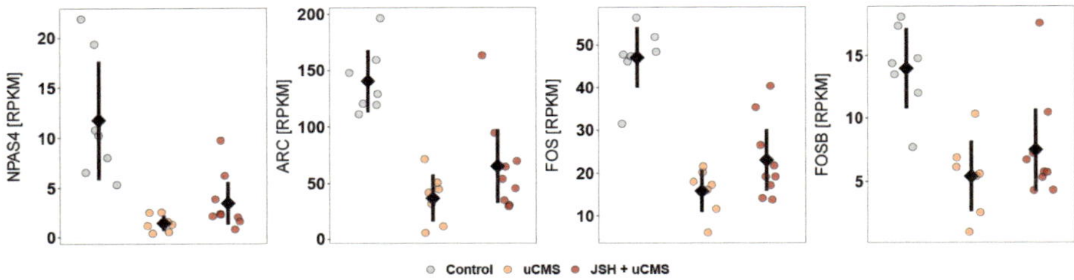

Figure 10.
Animal housing and stress protocols are described in ***Figure 4. Experimental details – Next Generation Sequencing:*** *RNA was extracted using the Ambion Magmax™-96 RNA isolation kit. In brief, cells were lysed (Qiagen Tissuelyzer™), nucleic acids were captured onto magnetic beads, washed, treated with Dnase and eluted in nuclease free water. RNA integrity and concentration were assessed using the Fragment Analyzer (Standard Sensitivity RNA kit, DNF-471, Advanced Analytical). Fifty nanograms of high quality RNA (RIN > 7) were used as input material for the NEBNext Poly(A) mRNA Magnetic Isolation Module and the NEBNext Ultra II Directional RNA Library Prep Kit (New England Biolabs). NEBNext Adaptors for Illumina were diluted 100 fold prior to cDNA ligation. Adaptor-ligated cDNA was amplified via 14 PCR cycles using NEBNext unique dual index primers (New England Biolabs). PCR products were cleaned up using AMPure XP Magnetic Beads (Beckman Coulter). Libraries were qualitatively and quantitatively assessed using the 1–6000 bp NGS kit (DNF-473, Advanced Analytical) and the Quant-iT PicoGreen dsDNA Assay kit, respectively. Final libraries yields were 40 nM, while fragment size were 350 bp. Libraries were normalized, pooled and clustered on the cBot Instrument using the TruSeq SR Cluster Kit v3 (GD-401-3001, Illumina Inc., San Diego, CA). The clustered flowcells were sequenced on a HiSeq 3000 using a read length of 84 bases in single-read mode, generating an average of 30 million pass-filter reads per sample.* ***Experimental details – RNA-Seq Data Processing:*** *Reads were aligned to the reference rat genome (Ensembl 84, http://www.ensembl.org) using the STAR Aligner (2.5.2a). Sequenced read quality was checked with FastQC (0.11.2, http,// www.bioinformatics.babraham.ac.uk/projects/fastqc/) and alignment quality metrics were calculated using the RNASeQC (1.18). Duplication rates of the RNA-Seq samples were computed and marked with bamUtil (1.u.11) and dupRadar (1.4), respectively. Cufflinks (2.2.1) was used to compute the reads per kilobase of transcript per million mapped reads (RPKM) as well as read counts. Normalization factors were calculated using trimmed mean of M-values (TMM) and subsequently reads were voom-normalized. Genes with RPKM values > 5 in at least one group were considered in the final analyses to ensure data quality. The Benjamini-Hochberg's method was used to correct for multiple testing, and only protein-coding genes with adjusted p value < 0.05 were considered as differentially expressed. Pathway analyses were carried out in Ingenuity.* ***Results:*** *Reduced expression of immediate early genes after stress in young adulthood. Next-generation sequencing of the PFC was used to quantify gene expression in controls (gray), uCMS alone (peach) and the double-hit group with JSH + uCMS (red). From all significantly different genes, only the most reliable with RPKM > 5 in at least one experimental group were eligible. There was a statistically significant reduction in the expression of Npas4 ($F(2,20) = 13.6$, $p = .0002$), Arc ($F(2,20) = 17.7$, $p < .0001$), Fos ($F(2,20) = 31.2$, $p < .0001$) and Fosb ($F(2,20) = 10.5$, $p = .0008$) in both stress groups compared to controls.*

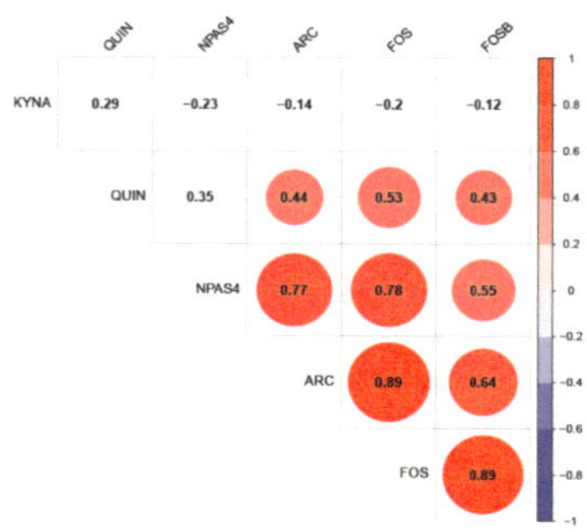

Figure 11.
Animal housing and stress protocols are described in ***Figure 4*** *while methods for TRYCAT profiling and NGS are described in* ***Figures 9*** *and* ***10****, respectively.* ***Results:*** *Correlation of immediate early gene (IEG) expression in the pre frontal cortex (PFC) with plasma levels of the neuroactive tryptophan catabolites (TRYCATs) kynurenic acid (KYNA) and quinolinic acid (QUIN) in 16 weeks old male Wistar Kyoto rats with and without stress exposure during adolescence and / or adulthood. Values represent Pearson's correlation estimate while the presence of surrounding circles indicates statistical significance at a false discovery level of $\alpha = .05$. Warmer colors mark positive correlations.*

to respond to incoming signals by changing its synaptic outputs [47, 48], was associated with decreased plasma levels of quinolinic acid (**Figures 8–11**, modified from [11]). This suggests that exposure to chronic stress can alter neurotransmission and connectivity in the brain via the kynurenine pathway, which modulates how the current situation is perceived and memorized. Ultimately, stress perception and memory influence how future events will be dealt with. Summed up, profiling of the tryptophan catabolites (TRYCATs) produced in the kynurenine pathway could represent an interesting biomarker for the balance of excitatory and inhibitory neurotransmission, plasticity and learning. TRYCATs may furthermore give insights into processes occurring in the PINE system in response to (chronic) stress, such as the presence of inflammatory processes.

4. Perturbations in the PINE network transition to disorder

The strong inter-connectedness of psychology, immunology, neurology and energy metabolism in the PINE network is very cost and time effective (**Figure 12**, modified from [11]). While the secretion of glucocorticoids as universal messengers in this system is seemingly unspecific, their pleiotropic effects on physiology are well regulated. The fine-tuning is implemented by complex combinations of ultradian GC levels at the event of challenge, the medium-term history of diurnal GC rhythmicity influencing enzyme and receptor expression levels, and the long-term evolved adaptations of PINE component connectivity incorporating the lifetime history of (stress) challenges. In acute stressful situations that decide over life and death, quick and pronounced stress responses are beneficial. However, sola dosis facit venenum and too frequent or much stress can be detrimental for health. The presence of a certain level of GC resistance is a common symptom of stress-associated medical conditions [49]. Resistance of PINE network components to their universal messenger would impede their effective communication. It is thus not surprising that GC resistance in the diseased state is featured with dysregulated immune processes, metabolism and cognition. Regarding the immune system, altered inflammatory signaling has been observed together with glucocorticoid resistance. Respiratory diseases, cardiac disorders, arthritis and inflammatory bowel disease all share a systemic low-grade inflammation associated with chronic stress exposure and altered GC signaling [50]. This chronic low-grade immune activation is not only discussed as feature of somatic disorders, but is as well studied as part of the pathophysiology of depression [51], which itself is a common comorbidity in the aforementioned disorders.

A further entry point for stress to alter the immune system functioning is via energy allocation. The role of bioenergetics has been shown for several aspects of immune system functioning and discussed in the context of therapeutic interventions [52]. Metabolism is not only influencing the activation and proliferation of immune cells [53] but mitochondria are also important for the inflammatory response [54] and regulation of the innate immunity via sensing of danger associated molecular patterns, the inflammasome and ROS-mediated oxidative signaling [55]. Limited mitochondrial capacities to respond to GCs would thus impede immune system regulation. In line with this mechanism, decreased mitochondrial functioning and evidence of slowed metabolism has been observed in patients with disorders where sterile, low-grade inflammation is a commonly observed symptom [56, 57]. Oxidative stress and the associated accelerated biological aging through damage is a likely cause for impaired mitochondrial functioning [29, 58]. Already in the prodromal phase of chronic stress exposure, strong cortisol responses to acute stressors were associated with oxidative stress, suggesting that stress exposure

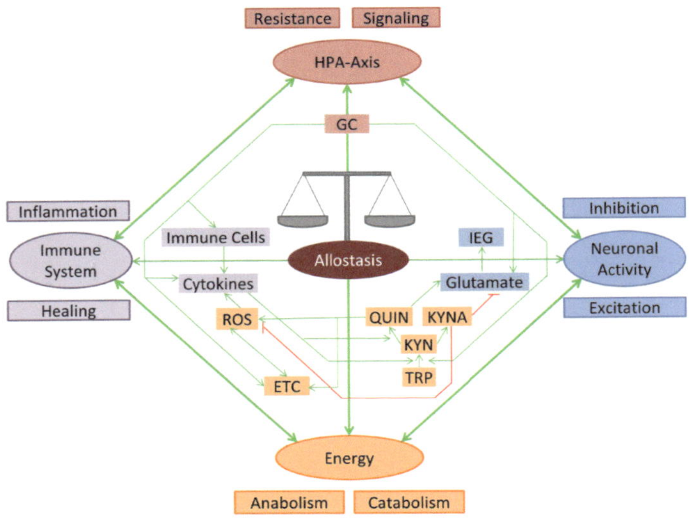

Figure 12.
Networking of the psycho-immune-neuro-energy system to balance allostatic load in response to stress.

promotes oxidative damage through frequent and sustained activation of the HPA-axis [59]. Interestingly, the excitatory neurotransmitter glutamate was shown to contribute to increased mitochondrial ROS production via a TSPO- and calcium-dependent mechanism, which adds to its excitotoxic potential [34]. In depressed patients, the loss of glial and neuronal cells in the PFC, amygdala and hippocampus has been observed [60–62]. Rumination of adverse thoughts in depression and strengthening of the fear-network in post-traumatic stress disorder could reflect enhanced memory recall based on increased hippocampal activity, which could explain the loss of cell density in later stages of the disease. Notably, timing and brain region seem to distinguish whether neuronal activity is beneficial or adverse. Increased hippocampal activity has been associated with stress and pathology, presumably given its sensitivity to compromised energy metabolism that might occur in the aftermath of chronic stress [63]. In contrast, synaptic weakening in the PFC has been associated with resilience to stress, which might be due to increased flexibility in the responsiveness to stress when response patterns are less fixed [48]. However, too few inhibitory outputs of the PFC to the hippocampus may lead to excess hippocampal activity and the resulting over-encoding of stress memory. Finding the right balance of excitatory and inhibitory signaling thus is essential for adequate stress responses and health. In psychiatric patients, this balance was reported to be disturbed [64]. Importantly, 'balance' does not mean a stable level, since the body needs to be able to respond to changes in its environment. As such, the system is never in balance during life but the ratio of excitation and inhibition oscillates following a diurnal rhythm alike glucocorticoids [65]. The need for rhythmicity in excitation and inhibition as well as GC levels is directly linked to the need of flexibility in the stress response system. Resiliency to stress is associated with a highly variable, adaptive capacity. This high degree of freedom in responsivity is key to evolutionary success in terms of fitting to constantly changing environments. Given that the specificity of glucocorticoid signaling is gained by its time and dose-dependency, attenuation in glucocorticoid rhythmicity in response to allostatic load would limit the fine-tuning of PINE network components. Decreased sensitivity or even resistance to GCs would limit their effective communication further. Likewise, the likelihood for persistency of taken adjustments would increase while the adaptive capacity of the PINE network would be reduced. This illustrates the clinical relevance of GC rhythmicity besides the role in sleep–wake regulation, plasticity or in the context of neurodegenerative disorders. Thus, monitoring the HPA-axis to effectively identify and treat many stress-related chronic illnesses begins to be part of the prevalent practice in the clinics. To fully access functionality, tracing of circadian rhythmicity and the cortisol-awakening response in addition to determination of the responsiveness of the HPA-axis is performed. The latter can be done using the Trier-Social-Stress-Test as challenge or by injecting dexamethasone, a synthetic glucocorticoid, to measure its suppressive effects on the HPA-axis. Patients with psychiatric disorders often show prolonged stress responses after challenge and less inhibition of ACTH and cortisol release when compared to healthy controls [66].

5. Conclusion

Taken together, altered GC signaling is a fundamental symptom in psychiatry that via its communicator role in the PINE network could explain certain other aspects of the diseased state like a pro-inflammatory milieu, compromised energy metabolism or changes in cognition. Whether the transition to disorder originates from this or the other components of the PINE network remains to be further elucidated. Presumably, disease development can not be explained by answering this linear hen-egg-problem but rather requires the joint integration of simultaneous alterations in all components. Therefore, no sequence of events that lead to disorder might be found, but rather patterns of local transitions [67]. These might differ from individual to individual based on the personal life experiences, genetic predisposition, and the surrounding environment. Moreover, the comorbidity of psychiatric and somatic disorders following chronic stress might suggests that maladaptive changes in the PINE network represent a shared prodromal stage in the etiology of these medical conditions. Our understanding of the mechanisms leading to pathology is far from complete and explanations to all facets of the disease remain to be discovered by holistic studies that consider the networking of psychology, immunology, neurology and energy metabolism.

Acknowledgements

The authors wish to thank their colleagues at Boehringer Ingelheim Pharma GmbH & Co KG Catherine Sweatman, Anne-Kathrin Ludwig, Margot Weiland, Sonja Diehl, Nadine Richter, Werner Rust, Nathan Lawless, Katrin Fundel-Clemens, Anna Lachenmaier, Tom Bretschneider, Silke Laack-Reinhardt, Yvonne Schneider, Sonja Hofbauer, Ralf Weber, Britta Gerth and Lukas Schmidt for their excellent support in performing the referenced own studies. We furthermore thank Alexander Karabatsiakis, Christina Böck, Iris-Tatjana Kolassa, Enrico Calzia and Peter Radermacher at Ulm University for their contributions to these studies.

Conflict of interest

The funding for the studies cited was provided by Boehringer Ingelheim Pharma GmbH & Co KG to provide a thesis project to V Nold. The company had no further influence on this work. V Nold and KA Allers are employees of Boehringer Ingelheim Pharma GmbH & Co KG.

Abbreviations

ACTH	adreno-cortico-tropic hormone
ATP	adenosine tri phosphate
CNS	central nervous system
CRH	corticotropin-releasing hormone
EAAT	excitatory amino acid transporters
ETC	electron transport chain
FKBP5	FK506 binding protein 5
GC	glucocorticoid
GR	glucocorticoid receptor
HPA	hypothalamus pituitary adrenal
HSP	heat shock protein
IDO	indolamine di oxygenase
KAT	kynurenine amino transferase
KMO	kynurenine mono oxygenase
LTP	long term potentiation
MR	mineralocorticoid receptor
mtDNA	mitochondrial desoxyribonucleic acid
NFκB	nuclear factor kappa-light-chain-enhancer of activated B cells
NMDA	N-methyl-D-aspartate
OXPHOS	oxidative phosphorylation
PFC	pre frontal cortex
PINE	psycho immune neuro energy
ROS	reactive oxygen species
TDO	tryptophan dioxygenase
TRYCAT	trypotophan Catabolite
TSPO	translocator protein

Author details

Verena Nold[1,2,3*] and Kelly Allers[1]

1 CNSDR Boehringer Ingelheim Pharma GmbH Co KG, Biberach, Germany

2 Clinical and Biological Psychology, Ulm University, Ulm, Germany

3 ADB Boehringer Ingelheim Pharma GmbH Co KG, Biberach, Germany

*Address all correspondence to: verena.nold@gmail.com

References

[1] T. Vos, A. D. Flaxman, M. Naghavi, R. Lozano, C. Michaud, M. Ezzati, et al. Years lived with disability (YLDs) for 1160 sequelae of 289 diseases and injuries 1990–2010: a systematic analysis for the global burden of disease study 2010. The Lancet, 380(9859): 2163–2196, Dec. 2012.

[2] A. J. Rush, M. H. Trivedi, S. R. Wisniewski, A. A. Nierenberg, J. W. Stewart, D. Warden, et al. Acute and longer-term outcomes in depressed outpatients requiring one or several treatment steps: A STAR*D report. *American Journal of Psychiatry*, 163(11): 1905–1917, Nov. 2006.

[3] R. Uher and A. Zwicker. Etiology in psychiatry: embracing the reality of poly-gene-environmental causation of mental illness. *World Psychiatry*, 16(2): 121–129, May 2017.

[4] Tasker, J. G., Di, S., and Malcher-Lopes, R. (2006). Rapid glucocorticoid signaling via membrane-associated receptors. *Endocrinology*, 147(12):5549–5556.

[5] Cain, D. W. and Cidlowski, J. A. (2017). Immune regulation by glucocorticoids. *Nature Reviews Immunology*, 17(4):233–247.

[6] Quatrini, L. and Ugolini, S. (2020). New insights into the cell- and tissue-specificity of glucocorticoid actions. *Cellular & Molecular Immunology*, 18(2): 269–278.

[7] Lorenz, O. R., Freiburger, L., Rutz, D. A., Krause, M., Zierer, B. K., Alvira, S., Cuéllar, J., Valpuesta, J. M., Madl, T., Sattler, M., and Buchner, J. (2014). Modulation of the hsp90 chaperone cycle by a stringent client protein. *Molecular Cell*, 53(6):941–953.

[8] Nold, V., Richter, N., Hengerer, B., Kolassa, I.-T., and Allers, K. A. (2020). FKBP5 polymorphisms induce differential glucocorticoid responsiveness in primary CNS cells – first insights from novel humanized mice. *European Journal of Neuroscience*.

[9] Sarabdjitsingh, R. A., Conway-Campbell, B. L., Leggett, J. D., Waite, E. J., Meijer, O. C., de Kloet, E. R., and Lightman, S. L. (2010a). Stress responsiveness varies over the ultradian glucocorticoid cycle in a brain-region-specific manner. *Endocrinology*, 151(11): 5369–5379.

[10] Kalafatakis, K., Russell, G. M., Harmer, C. J., Munafo, M. R., Marchant, N., Wilson, A., Brooks, J. C., Durant, C., Thakrar, J., Murphy, P., Thai, N. J., and Lightman, S. L. (2018). Ultradian rhythmicity of plasma cortisol is necessary for normal emotional and cognitive responses in man. *Proceedings of the National Academy of Sciences*, 115 (17):E4091–E4100.

[11] Nold, V., Sweatman, C., Karabatsiakis, A., Böck, C., Bretschneider, T., Lawless, N., Fundel-Clemens, K., Kolassa, I.-T., and Allers, K. (2019). Activation of the kynurenine pathway and mitochondrial respiration to face allostatic load in a double-hit model of stress. *Psychoneuroendocrinology*, 107:148–159.

[12] Spiga, F., Walker, J. J., Gupta, R., Terry, J. R., and Lightman, S. L. (2015). 60 YEARS OF NEUROENDOCRINOLOGY: Glucocorticoid dynamics: insights from mathematical, experimental and clinical studies. *Journal of Endocrinology*, 226(2): T55–T66.

[13] Jääskeläinen, T., Makkonen, H., and Palvimo, J. J. (2011). Steroid up-regulation of FKBP51 and its role in hormone signaling. *Current Opinion in Pharmacology*, 11(4):326–331.

[14] Fitzsimons, C. P., Herbert, J., Schouten, M., Meijer, O. C., Lucassen,

P. J., and Lightman, S. (2016). Circadian and ultradian glucocorticoid rhythmicity: Implications for the effects of glucocorticoids on neural stem cells and adult hippocampal neurogenesis. *Frontiers in Neuroendocrinology*, 41:44–58.

[15] Matosin, N., Halldorsdottir, T., and Binder, E. B. (2018). Understanding the molecular mechanisms underpinning gene by environment interactions in psychiatric disorders: The FKBP5 model. *Biological Psychiatry*, 83(10):821–830.

[16] Dhabhar, F. S., Malarkey, W. B., Neri, E., and McEwen, B. S. (2012). Stress-induced redistribution of immune cells—from barracks to boulevards to battlefields: A tale of three hormones – curt richter award winner. *Psychoneuroendocrinology*, 37(9):1345–1368.

[17] Filep, J. G., Delalandre, A., Payette, Y., and Földes-Filep, E. (1997). Glucocorticoid receptor regulates expression of l-selectin and CD11/CD18 on human neutrophils. *Circulation*, 96 (1):295–301.

[18] Caprio, M., Newfell, B. G., la Sala, A., Baur, W., Fabbri, A., Rosano, G., Mendelsohn, M. E., and Jaffe, I. Z. (2008). Functional mineralocorticoid receptors in human vascular endothelial cells regulate intercellular adhesion molecule-1 expression and promote leukocyte adhesion. *Circulation Research*, 102(11):1359–1367.

[19] Italiani, P. and Boraschi, D. (2014). From monocytes to m1/m2 macrophages: Phenotypical vs. functional differentiation. *Frontiers in Immunology*, 5.

[20] Bailen, N. H., Green, L. M., and Thompson, R. J. (2018). Understanding emotion in adolescents: A review of emotional frequency, intensity, instability, and clarity. *Emotion Review*, 11(1):63–73.

[21] VanTieghem, M. R. and Tottenham, N. (2017). Neurobiological programming of early life stress: Functional development of amygdala-prefrontal circuitry and vulnerability for stress-related psychopathology. In *Behavioral Neurobiology of PTSD*, pages 117–136. Springer International Publishing.

[22] Rose, S. P. (1995). Cell-adhesion molecules, glucocorticoids and long-term-memory formation. *Trends in Neurosciences*, 18(11):502–506.

[23] Sriram, K., Rodriguez-Fernandez, M., and Doyle, F. J. (2012). Modeling cortisol dynamics in the neuro-endocrine axis distinguishes normal, depression, and post-traumatic stress disorder (PTSD) in humans. *PLoS Computational Biology*, 8(2):e1002379.

[24] Fontanesi, F. (2015). Mitochondria: Structure and role in respiration. pages 1–13.

[25] Du, J., Wang, Y., Hunter, R., Wei, Y., Blumenthal, R., Falke, C., Khairova, R., Zhou, R., Yuan, P., Machado-Vieira, R., McEwen, B. S., and Manji, H. K. (2009). Dynamic regulation of mitochondrial function by glucocorticoids. *Proceedings of the National Academy of Sciences*, 106(9): 3543–3548.

[26] Liu, Y., Fiskum, G., and Schubert, D. (2002). Generation of reactive oxygen species by the mitochondrial electron transport chain. *Journal of Neurochemistry*, 80(5):780–787.

[27] Nunnari, J. and Suomalainen, A. (2012). Mitochondria: In sickness and in health. *Cell*, 148(6):1145–1159.

[28] Sies, H. (2015). Oxidative stress: a concept in redox biology and medicine. *Redox Biology*, 4:180–183.

[29] Jendrach, M., Mai, S., Pohl, S., Vöth, M., and Bereiter-Hahn, J. (2008). Short-

and long-term alterations of mitochondrial morphology, dynamics and mtDNA after transient oxidative stress. *Mitochondrion*, 8(4):293–304.

[30] Talabér, G., Boldizsár, F., Bartis, D., Pálinkás, L., Szabó, M., Berta, G., Sétáló, G., Németh, P., and Berki, T. (2009). Mitochondrial translocation of the glucocorticoid receptor in double-positive thymocytes correlates with their sensitivity to glucocorticoid-induced apoptosis. *International Immunology*, 21(11):1269–1276.

[31] Gerö, D. and Szabo, C. (2016). Glucocorticoids suppress mitochondrial oxidant production via upregulation of uncoupling protein 2 in hyperglycemic endothelial cells. *PLOS ONE*, 11(4): e0154813.

[32] Hara, Y., Yuk, F., Puri, R., Janssen, W. G. M., Rapp, P. R., and Morrison, J. H. (2013). Presynaptic mitochondrial morphology in monkey prefrontal cortex correlates with working memory and is improved with estrogen treatment. *Proceedings of the National Academy of Sciences*, 111(1):486–491.

[33] Picard, M., McManus, M. J., Gray, J. D., Nasca, C., Moffat, C., Kopinski, P. K., Seifert, E. L., McEwen, B. S., and Wallace, D. C. (2015). Mitochondrial functions modulate neuroendocrine, metabolic, inflammatory, and transcriptional responses to acute psychological stress. *Proceedings of the National Academy of Sciences*, 112(48): E6614–E6623.

[34] Gatliff, J., East, D. A., Singh, A., Alvarez, M. S., Frison, M., Matic, I., Ferraina, C., Sampson, N., Turkheimer, F., and Campanella, M. (2017). A role for TSPO in mitochondrial Ca^{2+} homeostasis and redox stress signaling. *Cell Death & Disease*, 8(6):e2896–e2896.

[35] Stobart, J. L. and Anderson, C. M. (2013). Multifunctional role of astrocytes as gatekeepers of neuronal energy supply. *Frontiers in Cellular Neuroscience*, 7.

[36] Rich, P. (2003). The molecular machinery of keilins respiratory chain. *Biochemical Society Transactions*, 31(6): 1095–1105.

[37] Virgin, C. E., Ha, T. P.-T., Packan, D. R., Tombaugh, G. C., Yang, S. H., Homer, H. C., and Sapolsky, R. M. (1991). Glucocorticoids inhibit glucose transport and glutamate uptake in hippocampal astrocytes: Implications for glucocorticoid neurotoxicity. *Journal of Neurochemistry*, 57(4):1422–1428.

[38] Lima, A., Sardinha, V. M., Oliveira, A. F., Reis, M., Mota, C., Silva, M. A., Marques, F., Cerqueira, J. J., Pinto, L., Sousa, N., and Oliveira, J. F. (2014). Astrocyte pathology in the prefrontal cortex impairs the cognitive function of rats. *Molecular Psychiatry*, 19(7):834–841.

[39] Slezak, M., Kandler, S., Veldhoven, P. P. V., den Haute, C. V., Bonin, V., and Holt, M. G. (2019). Distinct mechanisms for visual and motor-related astrocyte responses in mouse visual cortex. *Current Biology*, 29(18): 3120–3127.e5.

[40] Luarte, A., Cisternas, P., Caviedes, A., Batiz, L. F., Lafourcade, C., Wyneken, U., and Henzi, R. (2017). Astrocytes at the hub of the stress response: Potential modulation of neurogenesis by miRNAs in astrocyte-derived exosomes. *Stem Cells International*, 2017:1–13.

[41] Schousboe, A., Scafidi, S., Bak, L. K., Waagepetersen, H. S., and McKenna, M. C. (2014). Glutamate metabolism in the brain focusing on astrocytes. In *Glutamate and ATP at the Interface of Metabolism and Signaling in the Brain*, pages 13–30. Springer International Publishing.

[42] Bender, C. L., Calfa, G. D., and Molina, V. A. (2016). Astrocyte

plasticity induced by emotional stress: A new partner in psychiatric physiopathology? *Progress in Neuro-Psychopharmacology and Biological Psychiatry*, 65:68–77.

[43] Gibney, S. M., Fagan, E. M., Waldron, A.-M., O'Byrne, J., Connor, T. J., and Harkin, A. (2014). Inhibition of stress-induced hepatic tryptophan 2, 3-dioxygenase exhibits antidepressant activity in an animal model of depressive behaviour. *The International Journal of Neuropsychopharmacology*, 17 (06):917–928.

[44] Wu, H.-Q., Rassoulpour, A., and Schwarcz, R. (2006). Kynurenic acid leads, dopamine follows: A new case of volume transmission in the brain? *Journal of Neural Transmission*, 114(1): 33–41.

[45] Potter, M. C., Elmer, G. I., Bergeron, R., Albuquerque, E. X., Guidetti, P., Wu, H.-Q., and Schwarcz, R. (2010). Reduction of endogenous kynurenic acid formation enhances extracellular glutamate, hippocampal plasticity, and cognitive behavior. *Neuropsychopharmacology*, 35(8):1734–1742.

[46] Mattson, M. P. (2008). Glutamate and neurotrophic factors in neuronal plasticity and disease. *Annals of the New York Academy of Sciences*, 1144(1):97–112.

[47] Minatohara, K., Akiyoshi, M., and Okuno, H. (2016). Role of immediate-early genes in synaptic plasticity and neuronal ensembles underlying the memory trace. *Frontiers in Molecular Neuroscience*, 8.

[48] Wang, M., Perova, Z., Arenkiel, B. R., and Li, B. (2014). Synaptic modifications in the medial prefrontal cortex in susceptibility and resilience to stress. *Journal of Neuroscience*, 34(22): 7485–7492.

[49] Wright, R. J. (2009). Stress and acquired glucocorticoid resistance: A relationship hanging in the balance. *Journal of Allergy and Clinical Immunology*, 123(4):831–832.

[50] Mariani, N., Borsini, A., Cecil, C. A. M., Felix, J. F., Sebert, S., Cattaneo, A., Walton, E., Milaneschi, Y., Cochrane, G., Amid, C., Rajan, J., Giacobbe, J., Sanz, Y., Agust, A., Sorg, T., Herault, Y., Miettunen, J., Parmar, P., Cattane, N., Jaddoe, V., Lötjönen, J., Buisan, C., Ballester, M. A. G., Piella, G., Gelpi, J. L., Lamers, F., Penninx, B. W. J. H., Tiemeier, H., von Tottleben, M., Thiel, R., Heil, K. F., Järvelin, M.-R., Pariante, C., Mansuy, I. M., and Lekadir, K. (2021). Identifying causative mechanisms linking early-life stress to psycho-cardio-metabolic multi-morbidity: The EarlyCause project. *PLOS ONE*, 16(1):e0245475.

[51] Milaneschi, Y., Lamers, F., Berk, M., and Penninx, B. W. (2020). Depression heterogeneity and its biological underpinnings: Toward immunometabolic depression. *Biological Psychiatry*, 88(5):369–380.

[52] Faas, M. and de Vos, P. (2020). Mitochondrial function in immune cells in health and disease. *Biochimica et Biophysica Acta (BBA) - Molecular Basis of Disease*, 1866(10):165845.

[53] Pearce, E. L. and Pearce, E. J. (2013). Metabolic pathways in immune cell activation and quiescence. *Immunity*, 38(4):633–643.

[54] López-Armada, M. J., Riveiro-Naveira, R. R., Vaamonde-Garca, C., and Valcárcel-Ares, M. N. (2013). Mitochondrial dysfunction and the inflammatory response. *Mitochondrion*, 13(2):106–118.

[55] Chen, Y., Zhou, Z., and Min, W. (2018). Mitochondria, oxidative stress and innate immunity. *Frontiers in Physiology*, 9.

[56] Karabatsiakis, A., Böck, C., Salinas-Manrique, J., Kolassa, S., Calzia, E.,

Dietrich, D. E., and Kolassa, I.-T. (2014). Mitochondrial respiration in peripheral blood mononuclear cells correlates with depressive subsymptoms and severity of major depression. *Translational Psychiatry*, 4(6):e397–e397.

[57] Martn-Maestro, P., Gargini, R., Garca, E., Perry, G., Avila, J., and Garca-Escudero, V. (2017). Slower dynamics and aged mitochondria in sporadic alzheimer's disease. *Oxidative Medicine and Cellular Longevity*, 2017:1–14.

[58] Cui, H., Kong, Y., and Zhang, H. (2012). Oxidative stress, mitochondrial dysfunction, and aging. *Journal of Signal Transduction*, 2012:1–13.

[59] Aschbacher, K., O'Donovan, A., Wolkowitz, O. M., Dhabhar, F. S., Su, Y., and Epel, E. (2013). Good stress, bad stress and oxidative stress: Insights from anticipatory cortisol reactivity. *Psychoneuroendocrinology*, 38(9):1698–1708.

[60] Ongur, D., Drevets, W. C., and Price, J. L. (1998). Glial reduction in the subgenual prefrontal cortex in mood disorders. *Proceedings of the National Academy of Sciences*, 95(22):13290–13295.

[61] Bowley, M. P., Drevets, W. C., Öngür, D., and Price, J. L. (2002). Low glial numbers in the amygdala in major depressive disorder. *Biological Psychiatry*, 52(5):404–412.

[62] Lee, A. L., Ogle, W. O., and Sapolsky, R. M. (2002). Stress and depression: possible links to neuron death in the hippocampus. *Bipolar Disorders*, 4(2):117–128.

[63] Osborne, D. M., Pearson-Leary, J., and McNay, E. C. (2015). The neuroenergetics of stress hormones in the hippocampus and implications for memory. *Frontiers in Neuroscience*, 9.

[64] Sohal, V. S. and Rubenstein, J. L. R. (2019). Excitation-inhibition balance as a framework for investigating mechanisms in neuropsychiatric disorders. *Molecular Psychiatry*, 24(9): 1248–1257.

[65] Chellappa, S. L., Gaggioni, G., Ly, J. Q. M., Papachilleos, S., Borsu, C., Brzozowski, A., Rosanova, M., Sarasso, S., Luxen, A., Middleton, B., Archer, S. N., Dijk, D.-J., Massimini, M., Maquet, P., Phillips, C., Moran, R. J., and Vandewalle, G. (2016). Circadian dynamics in measures of cortical excitation and inhibition balance. *Scientific Reports*, 6(1).

[66] Ising, M., Depping, A.-M., Siebertz, A., Lucae, S., Unschuld, P. G., Kloiber, S., Horstmann, S., Uhr, M., Mller-Myhsok, B., and Holsboer, F. (2008). Polymorphisms in the FKBP5 gene region modulate recovery from psychosocial stress in healthy controls. *European Journal of Neuroscience*, 28(2): 389–398.

[67] Stapelberg, N., Pratt, R., Neumann, D., Shum, D., Brandis, S., Muthukkumarasamy, V., Stantic, B., Blumenstein, M., and Headrick, J. (2018). From feedback loop transitions to biomarkers in the psycho-immune-neuroendocrine network: Detecting the critical transition from health to major depression. *Neuroscience & Biobehavioral Reviews*, 90:1–15.